GET
THROUGH

MRCOG Part 2:
SBAs

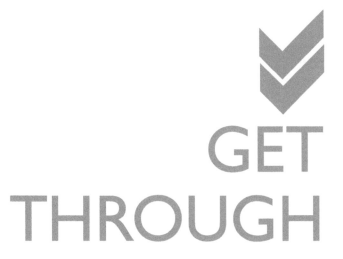

GET THROUGH

MRCOG Part 2:
SBAs

Rekha Wuntakal, MBBS, MD, DNB, MRCOG, DFFP
Consultant in Gynaecological Oncology and Gynaecology
Department of Obstetrics and Gynaecology, Queen's Hospital
BHR University Hospitals NHS Trust, London

Madhavi Kalidindi, MRCOG
Consultant Obstetrician and Gynaecologist
Queen's Hospital, BHR University Hospitals
NHS Trust, London

Tony Hollingworth, MB ChB, PhD, MBA, FRCS(Ed), FRCOG
Consultant in Obstetrics and Gynaecology
Whipps Cross Hospital, Barts Health NHS Trust
and
Senior Research Fellow
Centre for Cancer Prevention
Wolfson Institute of Preventive Medicine
QMUL, London

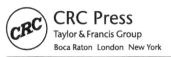

CRC Press
Taylor & Francis Group
Boca Raton London New York

CRC Press is an imprint of the
Taylor & Francis Group, an **informa** business

CRC Press
Taylor & Francis Group
6000 Broken Sound Parkway NW, Suite 300
Boca Raton, FL 33487-2742

© 2018 by Taylor & Francis Group, LLC
CRC Press is an imprint of Taylor & Francis Group, an Informa business

No claim to original U.S. Government works

Printed on acid-free paper

International Standard Book Number-13: 978-1-4987-2401-2 (Paperback)
978-1-138-48212-8 (Hardback)

Library of Congress Cataloging-in-Publication Data

Names: Wuntakal, Rekha, author. | Kalidindi, Madhavi, author. | Hollingworth, Tony, author.
Title: Get through MRCOG Part 2 : SBAs / by Rekha Wuntakal, Madhavi Kalidindi and Tony Hollingworth.
Description: Boca Raton, FL : CRC Press, [2018] | Includes bibliographical references and index.
Identifiers: LCCN 2018000007| ISBN 9781138482128 (hardback : alk. paper) | ISBN 9781498724012 (paperback : alk. paper) | ISBN 9781351058612 (eBook)
Subjects: | MESH: Obstetrics | Gynecology | United Kingdom | Examination Questions
Classification: LCC RG111 | NLM WQ 18.2 | DDC 618.10076--dc23
LC record available at https://lccn.loc.gov/2018000007

Visit the Taylor & Francis Web site at
http://www.taylorandfrancis.com

and the CRC Press Web site at
http://www.crcpress.com

CONTENTS

MATERNAL MEDICINE

Questions

THYROID

1. A 36-year-old woman with known hypothyroidism has been taking levothyroxine 100 micrograms once a day. Her most recent thyroid function tests performed 3 months ago were normal with a thyrotropin (TSH) of 2.5 mU/L. She has come to the early pregnancy unit with abdominal pain and a positive pregnancy test. Transvaginal ultrasound confirmed an intrauterine pregnancy.

   How would you advise with regards to her levothyroxine dosage?
   a. Decrease dose to 75 micrograms per day
   b. Decrease dose to 50 micrograms per day
   c. No change required
   d. Increase dose to 125 micrograms per day
   e. Increase dose to 150 micrograms per day

2. A 25-year-old woman known to have hyperthyroidism is going for radioactive iodine therapy. She has been trying to conceive for the last 6 months.

   How long should she avoid pregnancy after this treatment?
   a. 3 months
   b. 6 months
   c. 9 months
   d. 12 months
   e. 15 months

3. A 28-year-old para 1 woman at 40 weeks' gestation delivered a baby with a skin condition, diagnosed as 'Aplasia cutis congenita'. She is known to have hyperthyroidism secondary to Grave disease and has been on anti-thyroid medication throughout the pregnancy.

   Which one of the medications below is known to cause the above condition?
   a. Carbimazole
   b. Hydrouracil

c. Levothyroxine
d. Methythiouracil
e. Propylthiouracil

RENAL DISEASE IN PREGNANCY

4. A 38-year-old nulliparous woman with moderate chronic renal failure comes to the preconception clinic as she wishes to have a baby. She had renal transplantation 3 years ago and her recent creatinine is around 130 with estimated glomerular filtration rate (GFR) of approximately 45. She is currently taking prednisolone, mycophenolate, angiotensin-converting enzyme (ACE) inhibitors and aspirin. You have advised her to stop mycophenolate and to start another immunosuppressant.

   Which one of the immunosuppressant drugs would be contraindicated in pregnancy?
   a. Azathioprine
   b. Cyclosporine
   c. Hydroxychloroquine
   d. Sirolimus
   e. Tacrolimus

5. A 25-year-old para 1 woman at 30 weeks' gestation was brought in to the Obstetric day assessment unit with abdominal and back pains, vomiting and feeling unwell. Her observations are temperature 38.2°C, pulse 110 bpm, blood pressure (BP) 100/60 mm Hg, respiratory rate 18/min and oxygen saturations 98% on room air. On examination, she has suprapubic and right flank tenderness with 3+ leucocytes and positive nitrates on urine dipsticks. Foetal movements were good and cardiotocography was normal. You have admitted her and started broad spectrum intravenous antibiotics for acute pyelonephritis after doing the septic screen.

   What is the recurrence rate of pyelonephritis during the pregnancy?
   a. 5%
   b. 10%
   c. 15%
   d. 20%
   e. 25%

RENAL TRANSPLANTATION

6. A 35-year-old nulliparous woman with chronic renal failure had a successful renal transplantation surgery recently. She wishes to have children in the future and her GP has referred for preconception advice.

   What is the recommended time interval for conception after an allograft transplantation?
   a. 6 months

b. 12 months
c. 18 months
d. 24 months
e. 30 months

DERMATOLOGICAL CONDITIONS IN PREGNANCY

Skin

7. A 28-year-old woman at 32 weeks' gestation in her first pregnancy presented with a rash and itching on the abdomen, trunk, legs and hands. On examination, there were vesicles and bullae. A diagnosis of pemphigoid gestationis was made by the dermatologists after skin biopsies.

   Which one of the following statements is true about pemphigoid gestationis?
   a. Associated with other autoimmune diseases
   b. Most common dermatosis of pregnancy
   c. Not associated with any adverse effect on mother or foetus
   d. Rash usually begins in the abdomen with periumbilical sparing
   e. Recurrence in subsequent pregnancies is rare

8. A 30-year-old primigravida at 35 weeks' gestation with monochorionic diamniotic pregnancy presents with intense itching and rash on the abdomen. On examination there were erythematous papules and plaques in the striae gravidarum with umbilical sparing.

   The most likely diagnosis is which one of the following?
   a. Pemphigoid gestationis
   b. Polymorphic eruption of pregnancy
   c. Atopic eruption of pregnancy
   d. Prurigo of pregnancy
   e. Pruritic folliculitis of pregnancy

GASTROINTESTINAL TRACT (GIT) AND LIVER

9. A 34-year-old woman at 36 weeks' gestation was admitted with feeling unwell, vomiting and right-sided upper abdominal pain. On examination she was tender in the right upper quadrant with BP 140/90 mm Hg, pulse 90 bpm, temperature 37.6°C and protein 1+ in the urine. Her Hb was 128 g/L, platelets 160, white blood cell (WBC) count was elevated at 18, liver function was deranged with hyperbilirubinaemia and moderately raised alanine aminotransferase (ALT) and aspartate aminotransferase (AST). She was hypoglycaemic and clotting was mildly deranged with prolonged prothrombin time (PT) and activated partial thromboplastin time (aPTT). Renal function and liver scan were normal.

What is the most likely diagnosis?
a. HELLP syndrome
b. Pre-eclampsia
c. Cholecystitis
d. Acute fatty liver of pregnancy
e. Hepatic rupture

GIT AND LIVER

10. A 38-year-old primigravida at 36 weeks' gestation with dichorionic diamniotic twin pregnancy was diagnosed with acute fatty liver of pregnancy. She was stabilised and delivered by caesarean section.

    What is the risk of recurrence in subsequent pregnancies?
    a. 5%
    b. 10%
    c. 15%
    d. 20%
    e. 25%

INTRA-HEPATIC CHOLESTASIS OF PREGNANCY (IHCP)

11. A 26-year-old, nulliparous woman at 33 weeks' gestation presented with severe generalised itching that was worse at night and also present on the palms and soles. She was diagnosed to have intrahepatic cholestasis of pregnancy (IHCP) and was started on ursodeoxycholic acid and chlorpheniramine.

    Which one of the statements is true with regards to counselling women with IHCP?
    a. Ursodeoxycholic acid (UDCA) treatment improves foetal outcomes in women with IHCP
    b. There is good evidence that foetal risk is related to the maternal serum bile acid levels
    c. Liver function tests should be monitored twice weekly after the diagnosis of IHCP
    d. Risk of recurrence in subsequent pregnancies is about 90%
    e. Hormone replacement therapy should be avoided

SICKLE CELL DISEASE

12. A 28-year-old nulliparous woman with sickle cell disease (SCD) attends the preconception clinic for advice as she wishes to start her family. Her husband's haemoglobinopathy screen was normal, HbAA. You have reviewed her vaccination history and noted that she had haemophilus influenza type B,

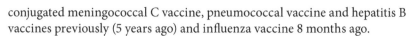

conjugated meningococcal C vaccine, pneumococcal vaccine and hepatitis B vaccines previously (5 years ago) and influenza vaccine 8 months ago.

Which one of the vaccines would you recommend her to have preconceptually?

a. Haemophilus influenza type b vaccine
b. Conjugated meningococcal C vaccine
c. Hepatitis B vaccine
d. Pneumococcal vaccine
e. Influenza vaccine

13. A 30-year-old nulliparous woman with sickle cell disease (SCD) attends your clinic for preconception advice. You have requested the following tests to assess for the chronic disease complications prior to stopping contraception.

    Which one of these screening tests is not indicated yearly?

    a. Pulmonary function tests
    b. Renal function tests
    c. Liver function tests
    d. Retinal screening
    e. Red cell antibody screening

BETA THALASSAEMIA

14. A 25-year-old woman with transfusion-dependent beta thalassaemia has been trying to conceive and undergoing ovulation induction.

    Which one of the statements is true with regards to young women with beta thalassemia major?

    a. Diabetes is the most common endocrine complication
    b. Hyperthyroidism is a known complication
    c. Desferrioxamine can be safely used throughout pregnancy
    d. Pneumococcal vaccine should be given annually
    e. Cardiac failure is the primary cause of death in more than 50% cases

THROMBOCYTOPENIA

15. A 26-year-old nulliparous woman at 36 weeks' gestation was diagnosed as having idiopathic immune thrombocytopenia (ITP). Her recent platelet count was 70×10^9/L.

    Which one of the following statements is true?

    a. Should be treated with immunosuppressants
    b. Regional anaesthesia is contraindicated
    c. Instrumental delivery is contraindicated
    d. Deliver by caesarean section at 37 weeks
    e. Neonatal thrombocytopenia occurs in 25% cases

SYSTEMIC LUPUS ERYTHEMATOSUS (SLE)

16. A 28-year-old para 1 woman with systemic lupus erythematosus (SLE) presents for a growth scan at 28 weeks' gestation. Foetal heart (FH) rate was 80–90 beats per minute and a foetal echocardiogram confirmed a second-degree congenital heart block (CHB).

    Which one of the following autoantibodies is associated with CHB in women with SLE?
    a. Anti-nuclear antibodies (ANA)
    b. Anti-double-stranded DNA antibodies (anti-dsDNA)
    c. Anti-Smith antibodies (anti-Sm antibody)
    d. Anti-Ro antibodies
    e. Anti-phospholipid antibodies (aPL)

VENOUS THROMBOEMBOLISM (VTE)

17. A 28-year-old nulliparous woman with anti-phospholipid syndrome (APS) and a previous venous thromboembolism (VTE) while on oral contraceptive pills is planning to conceive and seeks your advice.

    Which one of the options is the most appropriate with regards to her thromboprophylaxis in pregnancy?
    a. Higher dose of low molecular weight heparin (LMWH) antenatally and for 6 weeks postpartum
    b. LMWH antenatally and for 6 weeks postpartum
    c. LMWH from 28 weeks onwards and for 6 weeks postpartum
    d. LMWH postpartum for 10 days
    e. No need for thromboprophylaxis

THROMBOPHILIA SCREEN AND VTE RISK

18. A nulliparous woman had a thrombophilia screen requested by her GP because of the family history of VTE in her mother and sister.

    Which one of the thrombophilia defects is associated with the highest risk of VTE in pregnancy?
    a. Heterozygosity for factor V Leiden
    b. Prothrombin gene deficiency
    c. Homozygous factor V Leiden
    d. Protein C deficiency
    e. Antithrombin deficiency

DIABETES

19. A 25-year-old nulliparous woman with type 1 diabetes on insulin attends her first diabetic/antenatal clinic at 10 weeks' gestation. You have discussed diet, exercise, blood glucose monitoring and target blood glucose levels.

    Which one of the options is correct with regards to her capillary plasma glucose target levels?
    a. Fasting glucose 5–7 mmol/L
    b. Pre-meal glucose 4–7 mmol/L
    c. Fasting glucose below 5.8 mmol/L
    d. One-hour post-meal 7.8 mmol/L
    e. Two-hour post-meal 7.8 mmol/L

20. A 30-year-old nulliparous woman with poorly controlled type 1 diabetes attends a preconception clinic for advice. You have reviewed her recent HbA1c test results.

    At what HbA1c level should you strongly advise her not to get pregnant?
    a. Above 48 mmol/mol
    b. Above 58 mmol/mol
    c. Above 66 mmol/mol
    d. Above 76 mmol/mol
    e. Above 86 mmol/mol

GESTATIONAL DIABETES

21. A 30-year-old para 1 woman with a body mass index (BMI) of 38 and family history of diabetes attends antenatal clinic at 28 weeks' gestation. She was diagnosed with gestational diabetes 2 days ago when her glucose tolerance test was abnormal with a fasting glucose of 7.0 mmol/L and a 2-hour plasma glucose of 8.9 mmol/L.

    What is the most appropriate intervention in managing her gestational diabetes?
    a. Trial of changes in diet and exercise
    b. Diet + exercise + metformin
    c. Diet + exercise + glibenclamide
    d. Diet + exercise + insulin ± metformin
    e. Diet + exercise + insulin ± glibenclamide

Answers

1. d

EXPLANATION

In women with previously diagnosed overt or subclinical hypothyroidism taking levothyroxine prior to pregnancy, the dose should be increased initially by 25 micrograms daily once pregnancy is confirmed to compensate for the increased thyroxine demand and the increased plasma volume in pregnancy having a dilutional effect. Further increases may be required later in pregnancy. Thyroid function tests should be monitored every 4–6 weeks and further increases may be required to maintain optimal serum TSH levels (2.5 mU/L in the first trimester and 3 mU/L in the second and third trimesters). Once optimized, thyroid function tests need to be performed once in each trimester. After delivery, the pre-pregnancy dose should be restarted and thyroid function should be checked at 6 weeks postpartum.

Additional reading

Available at: https://stratog.rcog.org.uk/tutorial/
    diabetes-and-other-endocrinopathies/thyroid-and-pregnancy-5666
De Groot L, Abalovich M, Alexander EK et al. Management of thyroid dysfunction
    during pregnancy and postpartum – An Endocrine Society clinical
    practice guideline. *Journal of Clinical Endocrinology and Metabolism.*
    2012;97:2543–65.
Jefferys A, Vanderpump M, Yasmin E. Thyroid dysfunction and reproductive health.
    The Obstetrician and Gynaecologist. 2015;17:39–45. http://onlinelibrary.wiley.
    com/doi/10.1111/tog.12161/epdf
Nelson-Piercy C. *Handbook of Obstetric Medicine*, Fifth edition, 2015,
    Boca Raton: CRC Press.

2. b

EXPLANATION

Radioactive iodine is a commonly used treatment for hyperthyroidism, particularly Grave disease. Ideally women should be treated with surgery or radioactive iodine prior to becoming pregnant.

Radioactive iodine treatment is contraindicated during pregnancy, and pregnancy should be avoided for at least 6 months after treatment.

Additional reading

Available at: https://stratog.rcog.org.uk/tutorial/diabetes-and-other-endocrinopathies/thyroid-and-pregnancy-5666

De Groot L, Abalovich M, Alexander EK et al. Management of thyroid dysfunction during pregnancy and postpartum – An Endocrine Society clinical practice guideline. *Journal of Clinical Endocrinology and Metabolism.* 2012;97:2543–65.

Jefferys A, Vanderpump M, Yasmin E. Thyroid dysfunction and reproductive health. *The Obstetrician and Gynaecologist.* 2015;17:39–45. http://onlinelibrary.wiley.com/doi/10.1111/tog.12161/epdf

Nelson-Piercy C. *Handbook of Obstetric Medicine*, Fifth edition, 2015, Boca Raton: CRC Press.

3. a

EXPLANATION

Carbimazole and methimazole are associated with a congenital condition 'aplasia cutis congenita' in the foetus. This rare, reversible and benign condition is characterised by skin defects mostly on the scalp along the midline. The skin defects can also be seen in a symmetrical distribution peripherally on the trunk, face and limbs.

Though propylthiouracil is the preferred agent, carbimazole and methimazole are not contraindicated in pregnancy and need not be changed in women stable on these medications pre-pregnancy, as this complication is very rare.

Additional reading

Available at: https://stratog.rcog.org.uk/tutorial/diabetes-and-other-endocrinopathies/thyroid-and-pregnancy-5666

De Groot L, Abalovich M, Alexander EK, et al. Management of thyroid dysfunction during pregnancy and postpartum – An Endocrine Society clinical practice guideline. *Journal of Clinical Endocrinology and Metabolism.* 2012;97:2543–65.

Jefferys A, Vanderpump M, Yasmin E. Thyroid dysfunction and reproductive health. *The Obstetrician and Gynaecologist.* 2015;17:39–45. http://onlinelibrary.wiley.com/doi/10.1111/tog.12161/epdf

Nelson-Piercy C. *Handbook of Obstetric Medicine*, Fifth edition, 2015, Boca Raton: CRC Press.

4. d

EXPLANATION

Prednisolone, hydroxychloroquine, azathioprine, cyclosporine and tacrolimus are the immunosuppressant drugs that are safe to continue in pregnancy. Other immunosuppressants like mycophenolate mofetil and sirolimus, and cytotoxic agents like cyclophosphamide and chlorambucil are teratogenic and should be avoided in pregnancy.

ACE inhibitors and angiotensin II receptor blockers (ARBs) are antihypertensive, reduce proteinuria and offer renoprotection. But, they should be stopped preconceptually due to the risk of congenital malformations, and alternative antihypertensives like methyldopa, labetalol or nifedipine should be started.

Additional reading

Davison JM, Nelson-Piercy C, Kehoe S, Baker P. Renal disease in pregnancy. *Study group consensus views*. Cambridge, UK: RCOG Press; 2008. http://assets.cambridge.org/97819047/52592/frontmatter/9781904752592_frontmatter.pdf

Kapoor N, Makanjuola D, Shehata H. Management of women with chronic renal disease in pregnancy. *The Obstetrician and Gynaecologist*. 2009;11:185–91. http://onlinelibrary.wiley.com/doi/10.1576/toag.11.3.185.27503/epdf

Nelson-Piercy C. *Handbook of Obstetric Medicine*, Fifth edition, 2015, Boca Raton: CRC Press.

StratOG e-learning. https://stratog.rcog.org.uk/tutorial/renal-disease

5. d

EXPLANATION

Acute pyelonephritis complicates 1%–2% of pregnancies. It is more common in pregnancy due to the physiological dilatation of the upper renal tract. If there is no improvement within 48–72 hours, ultrasound of the urinary tract should be offered to exclude hydronephrosis, congenital abnormalities and renal calculi.

The recurrence rate for pyelonephritis is about 20%; hence, regular screening should be offered for asymptomatic bacteriuria for the remainder of the pregnancy.

Additional reading

McCormick T, Ashe RG, Kearney PM. Urinary tract infection in pregnancy. *TOG Review Article. The Obstetrician and Gynaecologist*. 2008;10:156–62.

Nelson-Piercy C. *Handbook of Obstetric Medicine*, Fifth edition, 2015, Boca Raton: CRC Press.

StratOG e-learnin. https://stratog.rcog.org.uk/tutorial/renal-disease

6. d

EXPLANATION

Pre-pregnancy advice for allograft recipients suggests 2 years of good general health is sufficient.

As per the European best practice guidelines, the following criteria are recommended for considering a pregnancy:

- Good general health for 12–24 months post-transplantation
- Good stable allograft function (serum creatinine preferably below 125 micromol/L)
- No recent episodes of acute rejection and no ongoing rejection
- Normotensive or minimal antihypertensive requirement
- Normal allograft ultrasound (no graft pelvicalyceal dilation)
- Recommended immunosuppressants at maintenance doses
- Prednisolone < 15 mg per day
- Azathioprine < 2 mg per day
- Cyclosporine or tacrolimus

Additional reading

Nelson-Piercy C. *Handbook of Obstetric Medicine*, Fifth edition, 2015, Boca Raton: CRC Press.
StratOG e-learning. https://stratog.rcog.org.uk/tutorial/renal-disease

7. a

EXPLANATION

Pemphigoid gestationis (PG) is rare dermatosis of pregnancy, occurring in 1:1700 to 1:50 000 pregnancies. It is an autoimmune condition and associated with other autoimmune diseases, particularly Graves disease. It can occur any time after the second trimester but rarely after delivery. The rash usually begins on the abdomen as urticarial papules and plaques around the umbilicus followed by the development of vesicles and bullae, extending to the trunk, extremities, palms and soles but with mucosal sparing. Skin biopsy and immunofluorescence are necessary to confirm the diagnosis.

Women should be managed jointly by an obstetrician and a dermatologist with emollients, topical corticosteroids and oral antihistamines in mild, pre-bullous cases and with oral prednisolone in the bullous phase of the PG. There is an association with foetal growth restriction; hence, antenatal foetal surveillance with serial scans is recommended.

Exacerbations and remissions are characteristic, with a postpartum flare occurring in about 75% of women. Recurrence may occur in subsequent pregnancies with earlier onset and increasing severity, and also with menstrual cycles and oral contraception.

Additional reading

Maharajan A, Aye C, Ratnavel R, Burova E. Skin eruptions specific to pregnancy: An overview. *The Obstetrician and Gynaecologist*. 2013;15:233–40.

Nelson-Piercy C. *Handbook of Obstetric Medicine*, Fifth edition. Chapter 13: Skin disease. 2015, Boca Raton: CRC Press.

8. b

EXPLANATION

Polymorphic eruption of pregnancy (PEP) is the second most common dermatosis of pregnancy, occurring in 1:160 to 1:300 pregnancies. Risk factors for PEP are nulliparity, multiple pregnancies or any other cause of overdistension of the abdominal skin in pregnancy.

Usual presentation is in the third trimester or immediately postpartum with no adverse effects on mother or foetus. Umbilical sparing is a typical feature of PEP. Recurrence is rare in subsequent pregnancies.

Additional reading

Maharajan A, Aye C, Ratnavel R, Burova E. Skin eruptions specific to pregnancy: An overview. *The Obstetrician and Gynaecologist*. 2013;15:233–40.

Nelson-Piercy C. *Handbook of Obstetric Medicine*, Fifth edition. Chapter 13: Skin disease. 2015, Boca Raton: CRC Press.

9. d

EXPLANATION

Acute fatty liver of pregnancy (AFLP) is a rare but potentially fatal condition due to multiorgan failure, especially if there is a delay in diagnosis and treatment. There is an association with primigravida, obesity, multiple pregnancies and male foetuses (ratio 3:1).

AFLP almost always occurs in the third trimester of pregnancy with gradual onset of nonspecific symptoms and liver dysfunction, and is usually associated with hypoglycaemia, hyperuricaemia, renal impairment and coagulopathy. It resolves completely postpartum with adequate supportive therapy.

Additional reading

Nelson-Piercy C. *Handbook of Obstetric Medicine*, Fifth edition. Chapter 11: Liver disease. 2015, Boca Raton: CRC Press.

StratOG e-learning. https://stratog.rcog.org.uk/tutorial/liver-and-gastrointestinal-disease/acute-fatty-liver-of-pregnancy-1554

10. e

EXPLANATION

The recurrence risk is approximately 25% and more likely if a woman is heterozygous for long-chain 3-hydroxy-acyl-coenzyme A dehydrogenase (LCHAD) deficiency, a disorder of mitochondrial fatty acid oxidation.

AFLP is associated with mutation of the gene related to LCHAD in 19% of cases. So, offspring of mothers should be screened for the common mutation E474Q.

Additional reading

Nelson-Piercy C. *Handbook of Obstetric Medicine*, Fifth edition. Chapter 11: Liver disease. 2015, Boca Raton: CRC Press.

StratOG e-learning. https://stratog.rcog.org.uk/tutorial/liver-and-gastrointestinal-disease/acute-fatty-liver-of-pregnancy-1554

11. d

EXPLANATION

Though UDCA improves pruritus, liver function tests and bile acid levels, there is no evidence to support or refute a beneficial effect of UDCA on the risk of foetal compromise and death. Also there is no robust evidence about the relationship between the foetal risks and the maternal serum bile acid levels.

Once IHCP is diagnosed, liver function tests should be monitored weekly until delivery and again at least 10 days after delivery. In women who have had IHCP, oestrogen-containing oral contraceptives should be avoided, but hormone replacement therapy should not be omitted.

Additional reading

Nelson-Piercy C. *Handbook of Obstetric Medicine*, Fifth edition. Chapter 11: Liver disease. 2015, Boca Raton: CRC Press.

Obstetric cholestasis. Green-top guideline No 43. April 2011. https://www.rcog.org.uk/globalassets/documents/guidelines/gtg_43.pdf

StratOG e-learning. https://stratog.rcog.org.uk/tutorial/liver-and-gastrointestinal-disease/obstetric-cholestasis-1544

12. d

EXPLANATION

Women should be given haemophilus influenza type b and the conjugated meningococcal C vaccine as a single dose if they have not received it as part of primary vaccination. The pneumococcal vaccine (Pneumovax, Sanofi Pasteur MSD Limited, Maidenhead, UK) should be given every 5 years.

Hepatitis B vaccination is recommended, and the woman's immune status should be determined preconceptually. Women with SCD should be advised to receive the influenza and 'swine flu' vaccine annually.

Additional reading

Eissa AA, Tuck SM. Sickle cell disease and beta thalassaemia major in pregnancy. *The Obstetrician and Gynaecologist*. 2013;15:71–8.

Management of sickle cell disease in pregnancy. Green-top guideline No 61. July 2011. https://www.rcog.org.uk/globalassets/documents/guidelines/gtg_61.pdf

Nelson-Piercy C. *Handbook of Obstetric Medicine*, Fifth edition. Chapter 14: Haematological problems. 2015, Boca Raton: CRC Press.

StratOG e-learning. https://stratog.rcog.org.uk/tutorial/haematological-disorders

13. e

EXPLANATION

The assessment for chronic disease complications in SCD should include the following:

- Screening for pulmonary hypertension with echocardiography should be performed if this has not been carried out in the last year. The incidence of pulmonary hypertension is increased in patients with SCD and is associated with increased mortality.
- Blood pressure and urinalysis should be performed to identify women with hypertension and/or proteinuria. Renal and liver function tests should be performed annually to identify sickle nephropathy and/or deranged hepatic function.
- Retinal screening. Proliferative retinopathy is common in patients with SCD, especially patients with HbSC, and can lead to loss of vision. There is no randomised evidence on whether routine screening should be performed or if patients should be screened only if they experience visual symptoms, but we recommend that women are screened preconceptually.
- Screening for iron overload. In women who have been multiply transfused in the past or who have a high ferritin level, T2* cardiac magnetic resonance imaging may be helpful to assess body iron loading. Aggressive iron chelation before conception is advisable in women who are significantly iron loaded.
- Screening for red cell antibodies. Red cell antibodies may indicate an increased risk of haemolytic disease of the newborn.

Additional reading

Management of sickle cell disease in pregnancy. Green-top guideline No 61. July 2011. https://www.rcog.org.uk/globalassets/documents/guidelines/gtg_61.pdf
StratOG e-learning. https://stratog.rcog.org.uk/tutorial/haematological-disorders

14. e

EXPLANATION

Young adults with transfusion-dependent thalassaemia develop hypogonadotrophic hypogonadism in 66%, diabetes in 20%, hypothyroidism in 10% and osteoporosis in 40% of cases. Cardiac failure is the primary cause of death in more than 50% of cases.

Iron chelating agents like deferasirox and deferiprone should be discontinued 3 months before conception and should be converted to desferrioxamine as the half-life is short and is safe for iron infusion during ovulation induction. It should be avoided in the first trimester due to lack of safety evidence, but can be continued after 20 weeks' gestation in low doses.

The pneumococcal vaccine should be given every 5 years, whereas haemophilus influenza type b and conjugated meningococcal C vaccine should be given as a single dose once.

Additional reading

Eissa AA, Tuck SM. Sickle cell disease and beta thalassaemia major in pregnancy. *The Obstetrician and Gynaecologist*. 2013;15:71–8.

Management of Beta Thalassaemia in pregnancy. Green-top guideline No 66. March 2014. https://www.rcog.org.uk/globalassets/documents/guidelines/gtg_66_thalassaemia.pdf

Nelson-Piercy C. *Handbook of Obstetric Medicine*, Fifth edition. Chapter 14: Haematological problems. 2015, Boca Raton: CRC Press.

StratOG e-learning. https://stratog.rcog.org.uk/tutorial/haematological-disorders

15. b

EXPLANATION

Thrombocytopenia is defined as a platelet count of $<150 \times 10^9$/L. The possible causes of thrombocytopenia in pregnancy include pregnancy-associated or gestational thrombocytopenia (75%), hypertensive pathology (15%–20%), immune causes (3%–4%) and others (1%–2%).

The diagnosis of ITP is one of exclusion. It can be associated with foetal and neonatal thrombocytopenia in 10% of cases. So, Ventouse delivery is best avoided as this may be associated with neonatal intraventricular haemorrhage if foetal platelets are low. Forceps can be used judiciously by experienced obstetricians. Caesarean section is only required for obstetric indications. Regional anaesthesia/analgesia is safe if platelet counts are $>80 \times 10^9$/L.

Close liaison with the haematology team is necessary in planning the management of this type of case. In mild cases, careful observation may be required but very low counts or significant bleeding risk may prompt treatment with corticosteroids or IV immunoglobulins or immunosuppressants.

Additional reading

Nelson-Piercy C. *Handbook of Obstetric Medicine*, Fifth edition. Chapter 14: Haematological problems. 2015, Boca Raton: CRC Press.

StratOG e-learning. https://stratog.rcog.org.uk/tutorial/haematological-disorders

16. d

EXPLANATION

CHB is a rare condition *in utero* which is permanent and associated with high mortality (15%–30%) and morbidity. CHB associated with neonatal lupus is considered to be a form of passively acquired autoimmune disease in which maternal autoantibodies to the intracellular ribonucleoproteins Ro and La cross the placenta and damage the foetal heart. CHB development is strongly dependent on a specific antibody profile to 52 kDa Ro.

In babies with Ro/La-positive mothers, the risk of transient neonatal cutaneous lupus is about 5% and the risk of CHB is about 2%. Not all Ro/La-positive mothers of neonates with CHB have SLE, but other associated conditions include Sjögren syndrome, Raynaud phenomenon or a photosensitivity.

Anti-Ro antibody is also called Sjögren syndrome A (SSA) antibody; and anti-La antibody as Sjögren syndrome B (SSB) antibody.

Additional reading

Nelson-Piercy C. *Handbook of Obstetric Medicine*, Fifth edition. Chapter 8: Connective-tissue disease. 2015, Boca Raton: CRC Press.

17. a

EXPLANATION

Women with VTE associated with either antithrombin deficiency or APS or with recurrent VTE (who will often be on long-term oral anticoagulation) should be offered thromboprophylaxis with higher dose LMWH (either 50%, 75% or full treatment dose) antenatally and for 6 weeks postpartum or until returned to oral anticoagulant therapy after delivery. These women require specialist management by experts in haemostasis and pregnancy.

Additional reading

Reducing the risk of venous thromboembolism during pregnancy and puerperium. RCOG Green-top Guideline No 37a. April 2015. https://www.rcog.org.uk/globalassets/documents/guidelines/gtg-37a.pdf

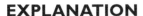

18. e

EXPLANATION

Antithrombin deficiency type 1 has the highest absolute risk of pregnancy-associated VTE in women with one or more symptomatic first-degree relatives.

Recent prospective and retrospective family studies support the view that deficiencies of the naturally occurring anticoagulants (antithrombin, protein C and protein S) are of greater clinical significance than heterozygous carriage of factor V Leiden or the prothrombin gene mutation. Recent studies have been consistent with a higher risk of pregnancy-related VTE in women who are antithrombin deficient or who are homozygous for factor V Leiden, the prothrombin gene mutation or are compound heterozygotes for factor V Leiden and the prothrombin gene mutation.

Additional reading

Reducing the risk of venous thromboembolism during pregnancy and puerperium. Green-top guideline No 37a. April 2015. https://www.rcog.org.uk/globalassets/documents/guidelines/gtg-37a.pdf

19. d

EXPLANATION

Advise **pregnant women** with any form of diabetes to maintain their capillary plasma glucose below the following target levels, if these are achievable without causing problematic hypoglycaemia:

Fasting: 5.3 mmol/L and 1 hour after meals: 7.8 mmol/L or 2 hours after meals: 6.4 mmol/L.

Advise pregnant women with diabetes who are on insulin or glibenclamide to maintain their capillary plasma glucose level above 4 mmol/L.

Target blood glucose levels preconception period

Advise women with diabetes who are planning to become pregnant to aim for the same capillary plasma glucose target ranges as recommended for all people with type 1 diabetes: a fasting plasma glucose level of 5–7 mmol/L on waking and a plasma glucose level of 4–7 mmol/L before meals at other times of the day.

Additional reading

NICE guideline NG3 – Diabetes in pregnancy: Management from preconception to the postnatal period. August 2015. https://www.nice.org.uk/guidance/ng3/resources/diabetes-in-pregnancy-management-from-preconception-to-the-postnatal-period-51038446021

20. e

EXPLANATION

Strongly advise women with diabetes whose HbA1c level is above 86 mmol/mol (10%) not to get pregnant because of the associated risks.

Explain to women with diabetes who are planning to become pregnant that establishing good blood glucose control before conception and continuing this throughout pregnancy will reduce the risk of miscarriage, congenital malformation, stillbirth and neonatal death. It is important to explain that risks can be reduced but not eliminated.

Additional reading

NICE guideline NG3 – Diabetes in pregnancy: Management from preconception to the postnatal period. April 2015. https://www.nice.org.uk/guidance/ng3/resources/diabetes-in-pregnancy-management-from-preconception-to-the-postnatal-period-51038446021

21. d

EXPLANATION

Offer immediate treatment with insulin, with or without metformin, as well as changes in diet and exercise, to women with gestational diabetes who have a fasting plasma glucose level of 7.0 mmol/L or above at diagnosis.

Offer a trial of changes in diet and exercise to women with gestational diabetes who have a fasting plasma glucose level below 7 mmol/L at diagnosis.

Offer metformin to women with gestational diabetes if blood glucose targets are not met within 1–2 weeks using changes in diet and exercise.

Consider glibenclamide for women with gestational diabetes in whom blood glucose targets are not achieved with metformin but who decline insulin therapy or who cannot tolerate metformin.

Additional reading

NICE guideline NG3 – Diabetes in pregnancy: Management from preconception to the postnatal period. April 2015. https://www.nice.org.uk/guidance/ng3/resources/diabetes-in-pregnancy-management-from-preconception-to-the-postnatal-period-51038446021

2 ANTENATAL CARE

Questions

ANTI D PROPHYLAXIS AND BLOOD PRODUCTS

1. A 30-year-old woman with a previous history of caesarean section and multiple uterine fibroids had a repeat elective caesarean section due to breech presentation. She had massive postpartum haemorrhage (PPH) secondary to uterine atony with an estimated blood loss of 3 L. She is RhD-negative and had transfusion of the group specific packed red cells, reinfusion of the salvaged red cells from the cell saver and also fresh frozen plasma (FFP), cryoprecipitate and platelets. The cord blood group was confirmed as RhD-negative.

   Anti-D prophylaxis should be administered in which one of the options, if she had the following blood products transfused?
   a. RhD-positive FFP
   b. RhD-positive cryoprecipitate
   c. RhD-positive platelets
   d. RhD-negative packed RBC
   e. Reinfusion of the salvaged red cells

MENTAL HEALTH

2. **A 20-year-old, nulliparous woman at 12 weeks' gestation attends her antenatal booking appointment. Which one of the following questionnaires was recommended to assess the mental health and well-being of the woman?**
   a. Depression identification questions
   b. Three-item Generalised Anxiety Disorder scale (GAD-3)
   c. Edinburgh Postnatal Depression Scale (EPDS)
   d. Patient Health Questionnaire (PHQ-9)
   e. Nine-item Generalised Anxiety Disorder scale (GAD-9)

3. A 28-year-old para 1 woman with history of bipolar disorder and previous postpartum psychosis attends her antenatal clinic appointment at 14 weeks' gestation.

What is her risk of developing postpartum psychosis?
a. 1 in 2
b. 1 in 4
c. 1 in 6
d. 1 in 8
e. 1 in 10

BREAST CANCER AND PREGNANCY

4. A 30-year-old nulliparous woman was treated for an early stage breast cancer 2 years ago and is currently taking tamoxifen. She wishes to conceive and attends clinic for your advice.

   Which one of the statements is most appropriate?
   a. Advise her to plan pregnancy
   b. Advise her to wait one more year before trying to conceive
   c. Advise her to stop tamoxifen and plan pregnancy
   d. Advise her to stop tamoxifen and wait for 3 months before trying to conceive
   e. Advise her to stop tamoxifen and wait for 6 months before trying to conceive

5. A 28-year-old nulliparous woman was diagnosed with an early stage breast cancer at 12 weeks of pregnancy.

   Her case was reviewed by the multidisciplinary team. What is likely to be their recommendation?
   a. Advise termination of pregnancy prior to surgical treatment
   b. Proceed with the surgical treatment
   c. Postpone surgical treatment until the second trimester
   d. Postpone surgical treatment until the third trimester
   e. Postpone surgical treatment until delivery

CHICKENPOX

6. A 28-year-old teacher was given varicella-zoster immunoglobulin G (VZIG) after a significant exposure to chickenpox at 24 weeks' gestation, as she was found to be seronegative on her booking bloods.

   How long should she be considered potentially infectious after exposure to chickenpox?
   a. 8–20 days
   b. 8–22 days
   c. 8–24 days
   d. 8–26 days
   e. 8–28 days

GENITAL HERPES AND HIV

7. A para 2, HIV-positive woman with low viral load and two previous normal vaginal deliveries was planning to have a vaginal delivery. She attends antenatal clinic at 28 weeks' gestation and says that she had a recurrence of genital herpes 2 weeks ago, which has now resolved.

   From what gestation would you advise her to take prophylactic daily suppressive acyclovir to reduce the risk of HIV transmission to the foetus?
   a. 28 weeks onwards
   b. 30 weeks onwards
   c. 32 weeks onwards
   d. 34 weeks onwards
   e. 36 weeks onwards

GENITAL HERPES

8. A nulliparous woman at 35 weeks' gestation develops primary genital herpes and an elective caesarean section was recommended by your consultant to reduce the risk of neonatal transmission of herpes simplex virus (HSV) at birth.

   What is the neonatal HSV transmission at birth?
   a. 10%
   b. 20%
   c. 30%
   d. 40%
   e. 50%

GENITAL HERPES AND PRETERM PREMATURE RUPTURE OF MEMBRANES (PPROM)

9. A para 1 woman at 33 weeks' gestation presents with preterm premature rupture of membranes (PPROM). She had a recurrence of genital herpes 3 days ago. On examination PPROM was confirmed, and the genital lesions are healing.

   What is the most appropriate management option?
   a. Steroids + erythromycin + oral acyclovir + delivery by caesarean section at 34 weeks
   b. Steroids + erythromycin + intravenous acyclovir + delivery by caesarean section at 34 weeks
   c. Steroids + erythromycin + oral acyclovir + consider induction of labour at 34 weeks
   d. Steroids + erythromycin + intravenous acyclovir + consider induction of labour at 34 weeks
   e. Steroids + erythromycin + oral acyclovir + delivery by caesarean section after completion of the two steroid injections

ANTEPARTUM HAEMORRHAGE

10. A 42-year-old, para 4 woman with pre-eclampsia comes to antenatal clinic at 34 weeks' gestation. She is asymptomatic with stable blood pressures on labetalol and the biochemical markers are normal. Growth scan confirmed foetal growth restriction. She is extremely anxious as she had abruption in her previous pregnancy that has led to an emergency caesarean section at 34 weeks' gestation.

    Which one of the risk factors has the most predictive value for abruption in this pregnancy?
    a. Advanced maternal age
    b. Multiparity
    c. Pre-eclampsia
    d. Foetal growth restriction
    e. Abruption in previous pregnancy

11. A 38-year-old para 3 woman with three previous caesarean sections has attended her first antenatal clinic appointment.

    What is her risk for placenta praevia in comparison to women with no previous caesarean sections?
    a. More than 5 times
    b. More than 10 times
    c. More than 15 times
    d. More than 20 times
    e. More than 25 times

CERVICAL CERCLAGE - SUTURE REMOVAL AND PPROM

12. A gravida 4 para 2 woman attends at 32 weeks' gestation with history of ruptured membranes. She had cervical cerclage placed at 13 weeks' gestation because of two previous preterm deliveries and one second trimester loss. She is well in herself with no signs of infection, not contracting, CTG is normal and PPROM is confirmed on examination. Scan confirmed normal growth, liquor and Doppler.

    Which one of the statements is true with regards to the timing of suture removal?
    a. Give steroids and remove suture immediately
    b. Give steroids and consider delayed suture removal for 24 hours
    c. Give steroids and consider delayed suture removal for 48 hours
    d. Give steroids and consider delayed suture removal for 72 hours
    e. Give steroids and remove suture when woman goes into labour

PRETERM LABOUR

13. A nulliparous woman was referred to the day assessment unit after an incidental finding of a cervical length of 18 mm with funnelling at 23 weeks' gestation by the sonographer. On speculum examination, no bulging membranes were seen. She had no previous cervical trauma or preterm deliveries.

    What is the most appropriate step?
    a. Offer expectant management
    b. Offer prophylactic vaginal progesterone
    c. Offer prophylactic vaginal progesterone and cervical cerclage
    d. Offer rescue cerclage
    e. Offer steroids and rescue cerclage

POLYHYDRAMNIOS

14. A nulliparous woman at 35 weeks was found to have polyhydramnios with an amniotic fluid index of 28 cm. Foetal growth was normal with no structural abnormalities; maternal glucose tolerance test, TORCH (toxoplasmosis, rubella, cytomegalovirus, herpes simplex) and parvo virus screen were negative.

    Which one of the options represents the incidence of idiopathic polyhydramnios?
    a. 10%–20%
    b. 20%–30%
    c. 30%–40%
    d. 40%–50%
    e. 50%–60%

15. A nulliparous woman at 35 weeks' gestation was referred for a scan as large for gestational age. The foetal growth was normal with no obvious foetal structural anomalies, but there was unexplained polyhydramnios with an amniotic fluid index of 29 cm.

    Which one of the statements is appropriate with regards her management?
    a. Offer amniodrainage to avoid preterm birth
    b. Commence indomethacin until delivery
    c. Deliver by caesarean section at 39 weeks
    d. Recommend induction of labour at 40 weeks
    e. Thorough neonatal survey should be performed

MULTIPLE PREGNANCY

16. A 30-year-old nulliparous woman with a monochorionic diamniotic (MCDA) pregnancy was diagnosed to have twin-to-twin transfusion syndrome (TTTS) at 18 weeks' gestation. There was significant discrepancy in the amniotic fluid volume with a maximum vertical pool of 1.8 cm in twin A and

polyhydramnios with maximum vertical pool of 10 cm in twin B. Both the bladders are seen and the Doppler studies are normal.

Which one of the options below represents the TTTS staging based on the Quintero classification system?
a. Stage 1
b. Stage 2
c. Stage 3
d. Stage 4
e. Stage 5

PERINEAL TEARS

17. You are seeing a 32-year-old para 2 woman at 16 weeks' gestation in the antenatal clinic. She had two previous normal vaginal deliveries, but sustained a third-degree tear during her second delivery. She is asymptomatic and is anxious about the risk of recurrence in this pregnancy.

    What is her risk of sustaining another third- or fourth-degree tear in this pregnancy?
    a. 1%–3%
    b. 5%–7%
    c. 10%–12%
    d. 15%–17%
    e. 20%–22%

FOETAL ANOMALIES

18. A 36-year-old para 3 woman attends day assessment unit after a growth scan for large for gestational age at 28 weeks' gestation. She had three previous normal vaginal deliveries and was low risk at booking. She declined first trimester screening, but had normal dating and anomaly scans. Growth scan showed polyhydramnios, small for gestation foetus with a double bubble sign, and she was referred to the foetal medicine unit by the sonographers.

    Which one of the aneuploidies is the foetus more likely to have?
    a. Down syndrome
    b. Edwards syndrome
    c. Klinefelter syndrome
    d. Patau syndrome
    e. Turner syndrome

NUCHAL TRANSLUCENCY

19. A healthy 36-year-old primiparous woman attended her dating scan at 12 weeks' gestation and was found to have a nuchal translucency (NT) of 4.5 mm. She is awaiting her first trimester screening results.

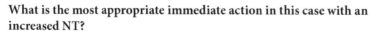

What is the most appropriate immediate action in this case with an increased NT?
a. Amniocentesis
b. Chorionic villus sampling
c. Ultrasound by a foetal medicine specialist
d. Foetal echocardiography
e. Non-invasive prenatal test

FIRST TRIMESTER SCREENING

20. A 40-year-old para 2 woman at 14 weeks' gestation attends antenatal clinic appointment. She had a normal dating scan and on the first trimester screening her pregnancy-associated plasma protein A (PAPP-A) was low at 0.33 MoMs (multiples of the median) and the free b-hCG was high at 2.4 MoMs.

    Which one of the aneuploidies is more likely than the others with these free b-hCG and PAPP-A levels?
    a. Trisomy 21
    b. Trisomy 18
    c. Trisomy 13
    d. Triploidy
    e. Turner syndrome

INHERITANCE PATTERNS

21. You are seeing a 30-year-old nulliparous woman in the antenatal clinic at 12 weeks' gestation with a family history of Duchenne muscular dystrophy. She is a known carrier and keen to know the likelihood of her children being affected.

    What is the likelihood of her children being affected?
    a. One in two chances of being affected
    b. One in four chances of being affected
    c. One in two chances of her sons being affected
    d. One in four chances of her sons being affected
    e. All daughters are affected

CYTOMEGALOVIRUS INFECTION (CMV) INFECTION

22. You are seeing a 35-year-old para 2 woman at 28 weeks' gestation with a small for gestation foetus in the antenatal clinic. She had TORCH screening and her cytomegalovirus (CMV) result was suggestive of a recent maternal infection.

    Which one of the following is most appropriate in woman with a recent primary maternal CMV infection?

a. Presence of IgM antibodies in the maternal serum indicates a recent primary infection
b. Risk of transmission is higher if CMV infection is acquired in the first trimester
c. High avidity of IgG antibodies is suggestive of a primary CMV infection
d. Primary maternal infection is associated with a 30%–40% risk of intrauterine transmission and foetal infection
e. Foetal infection is diagnosed when there are ultrasound markers of infection

SMALL FOR GESTATIONAL AGE (SGA)

23. You are seeing a nulliparous woman at 31 weeks' gestation in the day assessment unit after a growth scan. She was diagnosed with a small for gestational age (SGA) foetus at 28 weeks and having regular scans. The scan today confirmed foetal growth below the third centile with normal amniotic fluid index but abnormal umbilical artery Doppler with intermittent absent end diastolic flow. Middle cerebral artery and ductus venous Doppler scans are normal with no evidence of foetal redistribution.

    She had steroid injections 2 weeks ago when she presented with history of mild antepartum haemorrhage that was managed conservatively. Cardiotocogram is normal.

    What are the most appropriate recommended mode and timing of delivery?
    a. Caesarean section by 32 weeks
    b. Caesarean section by 34 weeks
    c. Induction of labour at 32 weeks
    d. Induction of labour at 34 weeks
    e. Induction of labour at 36 weeks

24. You were asked to see a para 2 woman at 36 weeks' gestation in the day assessment unit after a growth scan. Small for gestational age foetus was diagnosed at 34 weeks' gestation, and she is having scans every 2 weeks. The scan revealed growth along the third centile with normal amniotic fluid and positive end diastolic flow on umbilical artery Doppler, but with pulsatility index (PI) along the 95th centile. Middle cerebral artery Doppler scans are normal.

    What are the most appropriate recommended mode and timing of delivery?
    a. Caesarean section at 37 weeks
    b. Caesarean section at 39 weeks
    c. Induction of labour at 37 weeks
    d. Induction of labour at 39 weeks
    e. Induction of labour when Doppler scans show absent or reverse end diastolic flow

1. c

EXPLANATION

No anti-D prophylaxis is required if an RhD-negative woman receives RhD-positive FFP or cryoprecipitate.

The platelets should ideally be group compatible. RhD-negative women should also receive RhD-negative platelets. If RhD-positive platelets are transfused to a RhD-negative woman of childbearing potential, anti-D immunoglobulin should be administered. A dose of 250 IU anti-D immunoglobulin is sufficient to cover five adult therapeutic doses of platelets given within a 6-week period. This may be given subcutaneously to minimise bruising and haematomas in thrombocytopenic women.

Where an intraoperative cell saver (IOCS) is used during caesarean section in RhD-negative women, previously nonsensitised women and where cord blood group is confirmed as RhD positive (or unknown), a minimum dose of 1500 IU anti-D immunoglobulin should be administered following the reinfusion of salvaged red cells. A maternal blood sample should be taken for estimation of fetomaternal haemorrhage 30–40 minutes after reinfusion in case more anti-D is indicated.

Additional reading

Blood transfusion in obstetrics. Green-top guideline No 47. https://www.rcog.org.uk/globalassets/documents/guidelines/gtg-47.pdf

2. a

EXPLANATION

At a woman's first contact with primary care or booking visit and during the early postnatal period, consider asking the two depression identification questions and also using the 2-item Generalised Anxiety Disorder scale (GAD-2).

Depression identification questions: (1) During the past month, have you been bothered by feeling down, depressed or hopeless? (2) During the past month, have you often been bothered by having little interest or pleasure in doing things?

GAD-2 questions: (1) Over the last 2 weeks, how often have you been bothered by feeling nervous, anxious or on edge? (2) Over the last 2 weeks, how often have you been bothered by not being able to stop or control worrying?

If a woman responds positively to either of the depression identification questions, consider using the Edinburgh Postnatal Depression Scale (EPDS) or the Patient Health Questionnaire (PHQ-9) for full assessment, and similarly, if a woman scores 3 or more on GAD-2 scale, consider using GAD-7 scale for further assessment. If concerns, refer her to her GP or to a mental health professional if a severe mental health problem is suspected.

Additional reading

NICE Guideline (CG 192). Antenatal and Postnatal Mental Health. https://www. nice.org.uk/guidance/cg192/chapter/1-recommendations#recognising-mental-health-problems-in-pregnancy-and-the-postnatal-period-and-referral-2

3. a

EXPLANATION

Postpartum psychosis (PP) occurs in approximately 1–2 in 1000 women in the general population. Women with bipolar disorder have at least 1 in 4 risk of severe recurrence after delivery and need close contact and review during the perinatal period even if they are well.

The risk of PP is even higher in bipolar women with a personal or family history of PP, at greater than 1 in 2 deliveries affected by PP.

Additional reading

Di Florio A, Smith S, Jones I. Postpartum psychosis. *The Obstetrician and Gynaecologist*. 2013;15:145–50.

4. d

EXPLANATION

Women are generally advised to wait for at least 2 years after treatment for breast cancer before conception because of the risk of early relapse. The rate of disease recurrence is highest in the first 3 years after diagnosis and then declines, although late relapses do occur up to 10 years and more from diagnosis. Women with estrogen receptor positive disease should be advised that the recommended duration of tamoxifen treatment is 5 years.

Women on tamoxifen are advised to stop this treatment 3 months before trying to conceive because of the long half-life of the drug, and to have any routine imaging before trying to conceive to avoid the need for imaging during pregnancy.

Additional reading

Pregnancy and breast cancer. Green-top guideline No 12. March 2011. https://www.rcog.org.uk/globalassets/documents/guidelines/gtg_12.pdf

5. b

EXPLANATION

Surgical treatment including loco-regional clearance can be undertaken in all trimesters. Breast-conserving surgery or mastectomy can be considered, based on tumour characteristics and breast size, following multidisciplinary team discussion.

Radiotherapy is contraindicated until delivery unless it is lifesaving or to preserve organ function (e.g. spinal cord compression). If necessary, radiotherapy can be considered with foetal shielding or, depending on gestational age, early elective delivery could be discussed. Routine breast/chest wall radiotherapy can be deferred until after delivery.

Systemic chemotherapy is contraindicated in the first trimester because of a high rate of foetal abnormality, but is safe from the second trimester and should be offered according to protocols defined by the risk of breast cancer relapse and mortality.

Tamoxifen and trastuzumab are contraindicated in pregnancy and should not be used.

Additional reading

Pregnancy and breast cancer. Green-top guideline No 12. March 2011. https://www.rcog.org.uk/globalassets/documents/guidelines/gtg_12.pdf

6. e

EXPLANATION

Non-immune pregnant women who have been exposed to chickenpox should be managed as potentially infectious from 8 to 28 days after exposure if they receive VZIG and from 8 to 21 days after exposure if they do not receive VZIG.

Additional reading

Chickenpox in pregnancy. Green-top guideline No 13. January 2015. https://www.rcog.org.uk/globalassets/documents/guidelines/gtg13.pdf

7. c

EXPLANATION

Women who are HIV antibody positive and have a history of genital herpes should be offered daily suppressive acyclovir 400 mg three times daily from 32 weeks of gestation to reduce the risk of transmission of HIV infection, especially when a vaginal delivery is planned. Starting therapy at this earlier gestation than usual should be considered in view of the increased possibility of preterm labour in HIV-positive women.

There is some evidence that HIV antibody positive women with genital HSV ulceration in pregnancy are more likely to transmit HIV infection independent of other factors.

Additional reading

The joint BASHH and RCOG guidance. Management of Genital Herpes in Pregnancy. October 2014. https://www.rcog.org.uk/globalassets/documents/guidelines/management-genital-herpes.pdf

8. d

EXPLANATION

For women with primary HSV infection within 6 weeks of expected delivery, the risk of neonatal transmission is very high at 41%. Hence, caesarean section is the recommended mode of delivery for all women developing first-episode genital herpes in the third trimester, especially within 6 weeks of expected delivery.

Additional reading

The joint BASHH and RCOG guidance. Management of Genital Herpes in Pregnancy. October 2014. https://www.rcog.org.uk/globalassets/documents/guidelines/management-genital-herpes.pdf

9. c

EXPLANATION

When PPROM is encountered in the presence of recurrent genital herpes lesions, the risk of neonatal transmission is very small and may be outweighed by the morbidity and mortality associated with premature delivery.

In the case of PPROM before 34 weeks there is evidence to suggest that expectant management is appropriate, including oral acyclovir 400 mg three times daily for the mother. After this gestation, it is recommended that management is undertaken in accordance with relevant Royal College of Obstetricians and Gynaecologists (RCOG) guidelines on PPROM and antenatal corticosteroid administration to reduce neonatal morbidity and mortality and is not materially influenced by the presence of recurrent genital herpes lesions.

RCOG guidance on PPROM: Delivery should be considered at 34 weeks of gestation. Where expectant management is considered beyond this gestation, women should be informed of the increased risk of chorioamnionitis and the decreased risk of respiratory problems in the neonate.

Additional reading

Preterm prelabour rupture of membranes. Green-top guideline No 44. October 2010. https://www.rcog.org.uk/en/guidelines-research-services/guidelines/gtg44/

The joint BASHH and RCOG guidance. Management of Genital Herpes in Pregnancy. October 2014. https://www.rcog.org.uk/globalassets/documents/guidelines/management-genital-herpes.pdf

10. e

EXPLANATION

The predisposing risk factors for abruption include abruption in previous pregnancy, pre-eclampsia, foetal growth restriction, non-vertex presentations, polyhydramnios, advanced maternal age, multiparity, low body mass index (BMI), pregnancy following assisted reproductive techniques, intrauterine infection, premature rupture of membranes, abdominal trauma (both accidental and resulting from domestic violence), smoking and drug misuse (cocaine and amphetamines) during pregnancy, and first trimester bleeding/threatened miscarriage. Of these, the most predictive is abruption in a previous pregnancy.

Additional reading

Antepartum haemorrhage. Green-top guideline No 63. November 2011. https://www.rcog.org.uk/globalassets/documents/guidelines/gtg_63.pdf

11. d

EXPLANATION

Risk factors for placenta praevia include previous placenta praevia, previous caesarean sections, previous termination of pregnancy, multiparity, advanced maternal age (>40 years), multiple pregnancies, smoking, assisted conception and conditions that may cause deficient endometrium like uterine scar, manual removal of placenta, curettage, endometritis and submucous fibroid.

The odds ratio for placenta praevia in women with one previous caesarean section is 2.2, two previous caesarean sections is 4.1 and three previous caesarean sections is 22.4.

Additional reading

Antepartum haemorrhage. Green-top guideline No 63. November 2011. https://www.rcog.org.uk/globalassets/documents/guidelines/gtg_63.pdf

12. c

EXPLANATION

In women with PPROM between 24 and 34 weeks of gestation and without evidence of infection or preterm labour, delayed removal of the cerclage for 48 hours can be considered, as it may result in sufficient latency that a course of prophylactic steroids for foetal lung maturation can be completed and/or *in utero* transfer can be arranged.

Additional reading

Cervical cerclage. Green-top guideline No 60. May 2011. https://www.rcog.org.uk/globalassets/documents/guidelines/gtg_60.pdf

13. b

EXPLANATION

Offer prophylactic vaginal progesterone to women with no history of spontaneous preterm birth or mid-trimester loss in whom a transvaginal ultrasound scan has been carried out between 16+0 and 24+0 weeks of pregnancy and reveals a cervical length of less than 25 mm.

Offer a choice of either prophylactic vaginal progesterone or prophylactic cervical cerclage to women: with a history of spontaneous preterm birth or mid-trimester loss between 16+0 and 34+0 weeks of pregnancy and in whom a transvaginal ultrasound scan has been carried out between 16+0 and 24+0 weeks of pregnancy and reveals a cervical length of less than 25 mm.

Consider prophylactic cervical cerclage for women in whom a transvaginal ultrasound scan has been carried out between 16+0 and 24+0 weeks of pregnancy and reveals a cervical length of less than 25 mm and who have either: had preterm prelabour rupture of membranes (P-PROM) in a previous pregnancy or a history of cervical trauma.

RCOG guideline – The insertion of an ultrasound-indicated cerclage is not recommended in women without a history of spontaneous preterm delivery or second-trimester loss who have an incidentally identified short cervix of 25 mm or less.

Additional reading

NICE Guideline [NG 25]. Preterm labour and birth. November 2015. https://www.nice.org.uk/guidance/ng25/resources/preterm-labour-and-birth-1837333576645
Cervical cerclage. Green-top guideline No 60. May 2011. https://www.rcog.org.uk/globalassets/documents/guidelines/gtg_60.pdf

14. e

EXPLANATION

Polyhydramnios in the absence of maternal, foetal and placental aetiology is defined as idiopathic or unexplained, and is a diagnosis of exclusion. It accounts for 50%–60% of all cases of polyhydramnios.

It is associated with two- to five-fold increase in perinatal morbidity and mortality and linked with higher rates of malpresentation, macrosomia and primary caesarean sections.

Additional reading

Kharkanis P, Patni S. Polyhydramnios in singleton pregnancies: Perinatal outcomes and management. *The Obstetrician and Gynaecologist.* 2014;16:207–13.

15. e

EXPLANATION

Mild (25–29.9 cm) and moderate (30–34.9 cm) unexplained polyhydramnios:

- Perform serial scans and cervical length
- No benefit from induction of labour (IOL) for isolated/unexplained polyhydramnios. IOL only for maternal or foetal indications.
- Monitor progress of labour
- Watch for shoulder dystocia and postpartum haemorrhage
- Perform thorough neonatal examination and check patency of upper gastrointestinal tract with nasogastric tube

Severe (>35 cm) polyhydramnios – persistent or worsening or foetal abnormalities:

- Refer to a foetal medicine specialist
- Therapeutic amniocentesis/amniodrainage, if maternal discomfort/respiratory compromise from polyhydramnios or risk of preterm labour

Additional reading

Kharkanis P, Patni S. Polyhydramnios in singleton pregnancies: Perinatal outcomes and management. *The Obstetrician and Gynaecologist.* 2014;16:207–13.

16. a

EXPLANATION

TTTS complicates 10%–15% of MC pregnancies. Ultrasound examinations between 16 and 24 weeks focus primarily on detection of TTTS and after 24 weeks, the first presentation of TTTS is uncommon.

The Quintero classification system is as follows:

Stage 1 – There is a discrepancy in amniotic fluid volume with oligohydramnios of a maximum vertical pocket (MVP) ≤2 cm in one sac and polyhydramnios in the other sac (MVP ≥8 cm). The bladder of the donor twin is visible and Doppler studies are normal.

Stage 2 – The bladder of the donor twin is not visible (during length of examination, usually around 1 hour) but Doppler studies are not critically abnormal.

Stage 3 – Doppler studies are critically abnormal in either twin and are characterised as abnormal or reversed end-diastolic velocities in the umbilical artery, reverse flow in the Ductus venosus or pulsatile umbilical venous flow.

Stage 4 – Ascites, pericardial or pleural effusion, scalp oedema or overt hydrops present.

Stage 5 – One or both babies are dead.

Additional reading

Management of monochorionic twin pregnancy. Green-top guideline No 51. https://www.rcog.org.uk/globalassets/documents/guidelines/t51managementmonochorionictwinpregnancy2008a.pdf

17. b

EXPLANATION

The risk of sustaining a further third- or fourth-degree tear after a subsequent delivery is 5%–7%.

Additional reading

The management of third- and fourth-degree perineal tears. Green-top guideline No 29. June 2015. https://www.rcog.org.uk/globalassets/documents/guidelines/gtg-29.pdf

18. a

EXPLANATION

'Double bubble' sign appears when there is duodenal atresia causing distended stomach and the proximal part of the duodenum. This is associated with polyhydramnios, often appears in the late second trimester and is usually not detected at the anomaly scan.

Approximately half of the foetuses with duodenal atresia have associated abnormalities, including trisomy 21 (in about 40% of foetuses) and skeletal, gastrointestinal, cardiac and renal defects.

Karyotyping should be offered and in isolated duodenal atresia with normal karyotype the survival after surgery is more than 95%.

Additional reading

StratOG. RCOG e-learning resource – Core training – Antenatal care – Ultrasound scanning of fetal anomaly.

19. c

EXPLANATION

A nuchal translucency (NT) measurement ≥95th centile (≥3.5 mm) between 11 and 14 weeks' gestation is a strong marker for adverse pregnancy outcome. It is associated with an increased risk of foetal chromosomal anomalies, miscarriage, intrauterine death and various structural (especially cardiac) defects and rare genetic syndromes.

The prevalence of chromosomal defects increases exponentially with NT thickness. In the chromosomally abnormal group, about 50% have trisomy 21, 25% have trisomy 18 or 13, 10% have Turner syndrome, 5% have triploidy and 10% have other chromosomal defects.

Detailed anatomical ultrasound examination and echocardiography are recommended when the NT is elevated, and you should refer the woman for specialist scanning and counselling as the majority of structural anomalies are amenable to ultrasound detection. Non-invasive prenatal testing and invasive testing may not be required if the first trimester screening is low.

The majority of babies who achieve a normal scan and normal karyotype will have an uneventful outcome with no increased risk for developmental delay or other defects when compared to the general population.

Additional reading

StratOG. RCOG e-learning resource – Core training – Antenatal care –
  Ultrasound scanning of fetal anomaly. Fetal medicine foundation online
  resource – 11 to 13+6 weeks scan. http://www.fetalmedicine.com/synced/
  fmf/FMF-English.pdf

20. a

EXPLANATION

The level of free b-hCG in maternal blood normally decreases with gestation,
whereas the level of PAPP-A in maternal blood normally increases with gestation.

In trisomy 21 pregnancies at 12 weeks, the maternal serum concentration of free
b-hCG (about 2 MoM) is higher than in chromosomally normal foetuses, whereas
PAPP-A is lower (about 0.5 MoM). The difference in maternal serum free b-hCG
between normal and trisomy 21 pregnancies increases with advancing gestation,
and the difference in PAPP-A decreases with gestation.

In trisomy 18 and 13 maternal serum free b-hCG and PAPP-A are decreased. In
cases of sex chromosomal anomalies maternal serum free b-hCG is normal and
PAPP-A is low. In paternally derived triploidy, maternal serum free b-hCG is greatly
increased, whereas PAPP-A is mildly decreased. Maternally derived triploidy is
associated with markedly decreased maternal serum free b-hCG and PAPP-A.

Additional reading

StratOG. RCOG e-learning resource – Core training – Antenatal care –
  Ultrasound scanning of fetal anomaly. Fetal medicine foundation online
  resource – 11 to 13+6 weeks scan. http://www.fetalmedicine.com/synced/
  fmf/FMF-English.pdf

21. c

EXPLANATION

Duchenne muscular dystrophy is an X-linked recessive condition and is usually
only manifest in males. As males are hemizygous for X-linked genes, any male
with one copy of the X-linked recessive disease allele is affected. Females are

usually carriers and transmit the condition to one in two (50%) of their sons, and one in two (50%) of their daughters become carriers. Affected males pass the mutant gene to all their daughters who become obligate carriers, but not to their sons.

Other X-linked recessive conditions include Becker muscular dystrophy, Duchenne muscular dystrophy, Fabry disease, fragile X syndrome, haemophilias A and B, Hunter syndrome, ocular albinism, red-green colour blindness, testicular feminisation syndrome and Wiskott-Aldrich syndrome.

Additional reading

RCOG e-learning: StratOG – Core training – Antenatal care – Genetic disorders.

22. d

EXPLANATION

Diagnosis of primary maternal CMV in pregnancy should be based on seroconversion in pregnancy (i.e. *de novo* appearance of virus-specific IgG antibodies in the serum of pregnant women who were previously seronegative or on detection of specific IgM and IgG antibodies in association with low IgG avidity). The rate of foetal transmission appears to increase with advancing gestation – 34.8% in the first, 42% in the second and 58.6% in the third trimesters. However, sequelae in the offspring appear less severe if the transmission occurs later in gestation.

Primary maternal infection is associated with a 30%–40% risk of intrauterine transmission and foetal infection, with 20%–25% of those infected developing sequelae postnatally. Prenatal diagnosis of foetal CMV infection is based on amniocentesis performed at least 7 weeks after the presumed maternal infection and after 21 weeks of gestation.

Additional reading

Navti O, Hughes BL, Tang JW, Konje J. Comprehensive review and update of cytomegalovirus infection in pregnancy. *The Obstetrician and Gynaecologist.* 2016;18:301–7.

EXPLANATION

In the preterm SGA foetus with umbilical artery absent or reversed end diastolic velocity (AREDV) detected on Doppler prior to 32 weeks of gestation, delivery is recommended when DV Doppler becomes abnormal or UV pulsations appear, provided the foetus is considered viable and after completion of steroids. Even when venous Doppler is normal, delivery is recommended by 32 weeks of gestation and should be considered between 30 and 32 weeks of gestation.

In the SGA foetus with umbilical artery AREDV delivery by caesarean section is recommended.

Additional reading

The investigation and management of the small-for-gestational-age fetus. Green-top guideline No 31. January 2014.

24. c

EXPLANATION

In the SGA foetus detected after 32 weeks of gestation with an abnormal umbilical artery Doppler, delivery no later than 37 weeks of gestation is recommended.

In the SGA foetus detected after 32 weeks of gestation with normal umbilical artery Doppler, a senior obstetrician should be involved in determining the timing and mode of birth of these pregnancies. Delivery should be offered at 37 weeks of gestation.

In the SGA foetus with normal umbilical artery Doppler or with abnormal umbilical artery PI but end-diastolic velocities present, induction of labour can be offered but rates of emergency caesarean section are increased and continuous foetal heart rate monitoring is recommended from the onset of uterine contractions.

Additional reading

The investigation and management of the small-for-gestational-age fetus. Green-top guideline No 31. January 2014.

POSTPARTUM PROBLEMS (THE PUERPERIUM)

Questions

1. A 30-year-old para 1 woman presented 6 days after a normal vaginal delivery feeling unwell with a temperature of 38°C and pain in the right breast. On examination, there is a marked area of inflammation with tenderness.

   Which one of the following statements is correct with regards to mastitis?
   a. Group A streptococcus is the most common causative organism
   b. Mastitis may occur in the absence of bacterial infection
   c. Breastfeeding should be discontinued from the affected breast
   d. Mastitis commonly occurs in the lower left quadrant of the breast
   e. Ultrasound should be performed in all cases routinely

2. A 20-year-old, para 1 woman was brought in to the hospital 2 weeks after delivery as she has been tearful, irritable, with lack of interest in herself and her baby. She has not been eating or sleeping well, feels life is not worth living and has expressed thoughts of self-harming.

   What is the most appropriate immediate course of action?
   a. Admit to postnatal ward for observation
   b. Start antidepressant medication
   c. Refer to perinatal mental health team for follow-up
   d. Ensure urgent assessment by the perinatal mental health team
   e. Admit to mother and baby unit immediately

3. A para 1 woman was brought in by her family with postnatal depression 3 weeks after delivery. She had a caesarean section after a failed instrumental delivery and prolonged labour. She has been breastfeeding and wishes to continue to breastfeed.

   Which one of the antidepressant medication is safer during breastfeeding?
   a. Doxepin
   b. Fluoxetine
   c. Citalopram
   d. Escitalopram
   e. Sertraline

4. A nulliparous woman had a precipitous, spontaneous vaginal delivery and sustained a third-degree tear. At the end of the perineal repair in theatre, you have given diclofenac 100 mg suppository with consent. You would like to prescribe regular paracetamol and also a nonsteroidal anti-inflammatory drug (NSAID).

   Which one of the NSAIDs has the best safety profile?
   a. Ibuprofen
   b. Diclofenac
   c. Naproxen
   d. Meloxicam
   e. Fenoprofen

5. A para 2 woman with a body mass index (BMI) of 40, two previous caesarean sections and history of deep vein thrombosis at 33 weeks' gestation has taken her last dose of low molecular weight heparin (LMWH) at 6 a.m. the day before. Her elective caesarean section at 39 weeks was uncomplicated under combined spinal epidural (CSE) anaesthesia at 9 a.m., and the epidural catheter was removed at the end of surgery a few minutes ago, at 10 a.m.

   After what time can she have her LMWH injection?
   a. 10 a.m.
   b. 12 noon
   c. 2 p.m.
   d. 4 p.m.
   e. 6 p.m.

6. You have just delivered a 33-weeks preterm baby by caesarean section in good condition. Both mother and baby are stable.

   Which one of the statements is most appropriate with regards to the timing of cord clamping?
   a. Clamp cord as soon as possible
   b. Wait at least 30 seconds, but no longer than 1 minute
   c. Wait at least 30 seconds, but no longer than 2 minutes
   d. Wait at least 30 seconds, but no longer than 3 minutes
   e. Wait at least 30 seconds, but no longer than 4 minutes

7. A 30-year-old para 1 woman with gestational diabetes had a normal vaginal delivery. She has stopped her metformin and insulin after birth. At discharge, you have counselled her about the risk of developing diabetes and discussed lifestyle changes.

   Which one of the tests would you advise her to do postnatally?
   a. Fasting blood glucose at 6–13 weeks
   b. Fasting blood glucose after 13 weeks
   c. Oral glucose tolerance test at 6–13 weeks
   d. Oral glucose tolerance test after 13 weeks
   e. Oral glucose tolerance test after 24 weeks

8. A 32-year-old para 1 woman was admitted to the labour ward in spontaneous labour at 38 weeks' gestation. At delivery, she sustained a fourth-degree tear and was transferred to theatre for repair.

Which one of the following techniques is the most appropriate in the repair of a fourth-degree tear?
a. Interrupted sutures only to repair anorectal mucosa
b. Overlapping method to repair internal anal sphincter
c. Figure-of-eight sutures to repair the anal sphincter complex
d. End-to-end method to repair the partial thickness external anal sphincter tear
e. Overlap method to repair the partial thickness external anal sphincter tear

9. A 30-year-old nulliparous woman in a prolonged second stage of labour was delivered in theatre with ventouse. The baby was reviewed by the neonatal team, and there was a large well-defined swelling over the parietal bone of the foetal head with clear margins.

Which one of the following conditions is the most likely diagnosis for this swelling?
a. Caput succedaneum
b. Cephalhaematoma
c. Chignon
d. Subaponeurotic haemorrhage
e. Subgaleal haemorrhage

10. A 42-year-old para 3 woman with three previous normal vaginal deliveries and postpartum haemorrhage after her last delivery was induced at 39 weeks' gestation due to severe pre-eclampsia. She had an instrumental delivery for prolonged second stage and has consented for the active third-stage management.

What is the most appropriate immediate drug of choice?
a. Syntocinon 10 IU intramuscularly (IM)
b. Syntocinon 40 IU IV infusion
c. Syntocinon 5 IU intramuscularly
d. Syntometrine intramuscularly
e. Misoprostol 1000 micrograms rectally

11. You were asked to attend to a para 3 woman, who had a normal vaginal delivery 45 minutes ago in the midwifery-led birth unit and was transferred to the adjacent labour ward for retained placenta. She has moderate per vaginal bleeding, but is haemodynamically stable. IV access was secured and bloods were sent by the midwife.

What is your most appropriate immediate course of action?
a. Intra-umbilical vein injection of Syntocinon 10 units
b. Intramuscular injection of Syntocinon 10 units
c. Intravenous (IV) infusion of Syntocinon 40 units
d. Transfer to theatre for assessment under anaesthesia
e. Vaginal examination for assessment of the placenta

12. A para 4 woman with all previous normal vaginal deliveries and a big baby has just delivered spontaneously. She has consented for the active management of the third stage of labour and oxytocics were given at birth.

Active management of the third stage of labour reduces the risk of PPH by what proportion?

a. 20%
b. 30%
c. 40%
d. 50%
e. 60%

1. b

EXPLANATION

Mastitis is a painful inflammatory condition of the breast which may or may not be associated with infection. In lactating women, the primary cause of mastitis is milk stasis causing an inflammatory response that may or may not progress to infection. *Staphylococcus aureus* is the most common causative agent in infective mastitis.

Fever, malaise, breast pain and tenderness are the usual symptoms. It commonly presents as a tender, hot, firm, erythematous, unilateral swelling of the breast usually with a wedge-shaped distribution in the upper outer quadrant.

A penicillinase-resistant antibiotic, flucloxacillin or erythromycin (if allergic to penicillin) should be administered. Other measures include breast support, warm compresses and analgesics. Mothers must be advised to continue breastfeeding from the affected breast if possible. Failure to do so can worsen the condition by causing more 'congestion' and retention of milk in the affected duct.

If untreated, mastitis can lead to breast abscesses, necrotising fasciitis or toxic shock syndrome. Immediate referral to hospital is indicated if the woman is clinically unwell, has not responded to antibiotics within 48 hours, if the mastitis recurs or if there are very severe or unusual symptoms.

Any woman with a suspected breast abscess should be referred urgently to a general surgeon for confirmation of the diagnosis by ultrasound and for drainage of the abscess (by ultrasound-guided needle aspiration or surgical drainage). Complications of breast abscess include early weaning, inability to breastfeed in the future and the need for resection.

Additional reading

Bacterial sepsis following pregnancy. Green-top guideline No 64b. https://www.rcog.org.uk/globalassets/documents/guidelines/gtg_64b.pdf

NICE clinical knowledge summary guidance on mastitis and breast abscess. http://cks.nice.org.uk/mastitis-and-breast-abscess#!topicsummary

2. d

EXPLANATION

The diagnosis is severe postnatal depression with thoughts of self-harm/suicidal ideations. She should be referred immediately to the perinatal mental health team (local psychiatric liaison teams out of hours) for urgent assessment, admission and initiation of treatment with antidepressant medication along with the supportive psychotherapy.

Additional reading

Oates M. Postnatal affective disorders. Part 1: An introduction. *The Obstetrician and Gynaecologist.* 2008;10:145–50.

Oates M. Postnatal affective disorders. Part 2: Prevention and management. *The Obstetrician and Gynaecologist.* 2008;10:231–5.

RCOG Good Practice Guidance 14 - Management of women with mental health issues during pregnancy and the postnatal period. https://www.rcog.org.uk/globalassets/documents/guidelines/ managementwomenmentalhealthgoodpractice14.pdf

3. e

EXPLANATION

Breastfeeding is an individual decision for each woman, and clinicians should support women in their choice and be mindful that taking prescribed psychotropic medication is not routinely a contraindication to commencing or continuing breastfeeding.

Avoid doxepin for treatment of depression in women who are breastfeeding. If initiating selective serotonin reuptake inhibitor (SSRI) treatment in breastfeeding, then fluoxetine, citalopram and escitalopram should be avoided if possible. Imipramine, nortriptyline and sertraline are present at relatively low levels in breast milk.

Additional reading

NICE Guideline (CG 192) – Antenatal and Postnatal Mental Health.

Scottish Intercollegiate Guidelines Network (SIGN) – Management of perinatal mood disorders.

4. a

EXPLANATION

NSAIDs constitute useful postpartum analgesics with a low incidence of adverse effects in the healthy population. Ibuprofen is the first-line NSAID and has the best safety profile.

The National Institute for Health and Care Excellence (NICE) guidelines recommend the use of NSAIDs in the postpartum period for perineal pain when paracetamol provides insufficient relief of symptoms. A meta-analysis has shown that rectal NSAIDs given after episiotomy are associated with less discomfort in the 24 hours after delivery.

Additional reading

Wiles KS, Banerjee A. Acute kidney injury in pregnancy and the use of non-steroidal anti-inflammatory drugs. *The Obstetrician and Gynaecologist.* 2016;18:127–35.

5. c

EXPLANATION

LMWH should not be given for 4 hours after the use of spinal anaesthesia or after the epidural catheter has been removed, and the epidural catheter should not be removed within 12 hours of the most recent injection.

Additional reading

Reducing the risk of venous thromboembolism during pregnancy and puerperium. Green-top guideline No 37a. https://www.rcog.org.uk/globalassets/documents/guidelines/gtg-37a.pdf

Thromboembolic disease in pregnancy and puerperium. Green-top guideline No 37b. April 2015. https://www.rcog.org.uk/globalassets/documents/guidelines/gtg-37b.pdf

6. d

EXPLANATION

If a preterm baby needs to be moved away from the mother for resuscitation, or there is significant maternal bleeding: consider milking the cord and clamp the cord as soon as possible.

Wait at least 30 seconds, but no longer than 3 minutes, before clamping the cord of preterm babies if the mother and baby are stable.

Position the baby at or below the level of the placenta before clamping the cord.

Additional reading

NICE Guideline [NG 25] – Preterm labour and birth. November 2015. https://www.nice.org.uk/guidance/ng25/resources/preterm-labour-and-birth-1837333576645

7. a

EXPLANATION

Gestational diabetes is one of the strongest risk factors for the subsequent development of type 2 diabetes: up to 50% of women diagnosed with gestational diabetes develop type 2 diabetes within 5 years of the birth.

For women who were diagnosed with gestational diabetes and whose blood glucose levels returned to normal after the birth: Offer lifestyle advice (including weight control, diet and exercise) and a fasting plasma glucose test 6–13 weeks after the birth to exclude diabetes. (For practical reasons this might take place at the 6-week postnatal check.)

If a fasting plasma glucose test has not been performed by 13 weeks, offer a fasting plasma glucose test, or an HbA1c test if a fasting plasma glucose test is not possible, after 13 weeks.

Do not routinely offer a 75 g 2-hour oral glucose tolerance test (OGTT).

Additional reading

NICE guideline NG3 – Diabetes in pregnancy: Management from preconception to the postnatal period. https://www.nice.org.uk/guidance/ng3/resources/diabetes-in-pregnancy-management-from-preconception-to-the-postnatal-period-51038446021

8. d

EXPLANATION

The torn anorectal mucosa should be repaired with sutures using either the continuous or interrupted technique. Figure-of-eight sutures should be avoided during the repair of obstetric anal sphincter injuries (OASIS) because they are haemostatic in nature and may cause tissue ischaemia.

Where the torn internal anal sphincter (IAS) can be identified, it is advisable to repair this separately with interrupted or mattress sutures without any attempt to overlap the IAS.

For repair of a full-thickness external anal sphincter (EAS) tear, either an overlapping or an end-to-end (approximation) method can be used with equivalent outcomes. For partial-thickness (all 3a and some 3b) tears, an end-to-end technique should be used.

Additional reading

The management of third- and fourth-degree perineal tears. Green-top guideline No. 29. June 2015. https://www.rcog.org.uk/globalassets/documents/guidelines/gtg-29.pdf

9. b

EXPLANATION

Cephalhaematoma is a subperiosteal collection of blood between the periosteum and the skull due to rupture of blood vessels and may be associated with skull fracture. It is well defined as the hematoma is confined to the subperiosteal space with clear delineation of the suture lines. It is most commonly parietal, but occasionally it may be seen on the occipital bone.

Caput succedaneum is a subcutaneous, extraperiosteal serosanguineous fluid collection and is caused by the pressure of the presenting part against the dilating cervix. It extends across the midline and over the suture lines with poorly defined margins. Chignon is a temporary swelling on the baby's head at the ventouse cup application site.

Subgaleal or subaponeurotic haemorrhage/haematoma develops when there is bleeding between the periosteum and the scalp galea aponeurosis. A fluctuant boggy mass develops over the scalp gradually across the whole skull, crosses suture lines and is usually secondary to multiple attempts at ventouse delivery.

Additional reading

StratOG e-learning resource: Core training – Postpartum and neonatal problems – Assessment of the newborn and common neonatal problems.

10. a

EXPLANATION

Active management of the third stage involves

- Routine use of uterotonic drugs
- Delayed clamping and cutting of the cord (Do not clamp the cord earlier than 1 minute from the birth of the baby unless there is concern about foetal distress)
- Controlled cord traction after signs of separation of the placenta

For active management, administer 10 IU of oxytocin IM with the birth of the anterior shoulder or immediately after the birth of the baby and before the cord is clamped and cut. Oxytocin is preferred to syntometrine due to fewer side effects.

Syntometrine (Alliance) may be used in the absence of hypertension (for instance, antenatal low haemoglobin) as it reduces the risk of minor postpartum haemorrhage (PPH) (500–1000 mL) but increases vomiting.

Misoprostol is not as effective as oxytocin, but it may be used when the latter is not available, such as in the home-birth setting.

Additional reading

NICE clinical guidance CG 190: Intrapartum care for healthy women and babies. December 2014. https://www.nice.org.uk/guidance/cg190
Prevention and management of postpartum haemorrhage. Green-top guideline No 52. April 2011. https://www.rcog.org.uk/globalassets/documents/guidelines/gt52postpartumhaemorrhage0411.pdf

11. e

EXPLANATION

If the placenta is retained and IV access secured, then vaginal examination should be undertaken to assess the need for manual removal of placenta.

Do not use umbilical vein agents or IV oxytocin agents routinely to deliver a retained placenta. Give IV oxytocin agents if bleeding is excessive and the placenta is retained; and make the necessary arrangements for uterine exploration in theatre under anaesthesia.

Additional reading

NICE clinical guidance CG 190: Intrapartum care for healthy women and babies. December 2014. https://www.nice.org.uk/guidance/cg190

12. e

EXPLANATION

Active management of the third stage of labour lowers maternal blood loss and reduces the risk of PPH. Prophylactic oxytocics should be offered routinely in the management of the third stage of labour in all women as they reduce the risk of PPH by about 60%.

Additional reading

Prevention and management of postpartum haemorrhage. Green-top guideline No 52. April 2011. https://www.rcog.org.uk/globalassets/documents/guidelines/gt52postpartumhaemorrhage0411.pdf

ETHICS AND LEGAL ISSUES AND CONSENT

Questions

1. A 12-year-old girl was brought in to the hospital with severe lower abdominal pain and was diagnosed to have hematometrocolpos after examination and investigations. Surgical management with hymenotomy and drainage was recommended the same day by the consultant on call, who gave a clear explanation of the procedure, reasons, implications and risks. The young girl instantly declined as she was too scared of the operation, but later agreed after her mother and stepfather calmed her down.

   From which one of the following options is it most appropriate for you to obtain consent?
   a. Consent from the patient alone
   b. Consent from the mother alone
   c. Consent from the patient and mother
   d. Consent from the patient and stepfather
   e. Consent from both parents

2. A 15-year-old girl accompanied by her friend presents to the emergency gynaecology unit with crampy lower abdominal pain and vaginal bleeding. Her observations were stable. Her last menstrual period was 7 weeks ago and the urine pregnancy test was positive. Ultrasound performed showed missed miscarriage. After discussing the options, she opted for surgical management of miscarriage and requests you to keep this confidential as her parents are not aware.
   a. You can proceed with the girl's consent, as the mother's consent is not necessary
   b. Mother's consent is necessary and you encourage her to inform her mother
   c. Mother's consent is necessary and you would like to inform with the patient's consent
   d. You can proceed with the girl's consent, but you need to inform social services
   e. You can proceed with the girl's consent after obtaining a second consultant approval

3. A 30-year-old nulliparous woman had an uncomplicated forceps delivery at term for prolonged second stage and an abnormal cardiotocogram (CTG). The baby was born in poor condition, and developed seizures secondary to hypoxic ischemic encephalopathy after birth. The baby is now 5 years old and has severe cerebral palsy.

Until what age can the baby bring a claim attributing the cerebral palsy to the suboptimal intrapartum care or for medical negligence?
   a. Three years from the date of knowledge
   b. Five years from the date of knowledge
   c. Three years from the 18th birthday
   d. Five years from the 18th birthday
   e. No age limit

4. A 39-year-old para 1 woman with two previous normal vaginal deliveries presents in spontaneous labour at 38 weeks' gestation. She developed gestational hypertension at 35 weeks, though is currently asymptomatic with stable blood pressures on antihypertensives. She had good progress in labour, but the CTG became abnormal at 8 cm cervical dilatation with a pH of 7.19 on foetal blood sampling. She has declined caesarean section as she does not want to have an operation. She had similar problems in her last pregnancy but had a normal delivery with a healthy baby. She understands the risks, and you have clearly documented your discussions with her.

You are the consultant in charge. What is the most appropriate management option?
   a. Discuss with her partner in order to influence her decision
   b. Obtain a second opinion from another consultant
   c. Respect her wishes and review appropriately
   d. Obtain a second opinion from the psychiatry team to assess capacity
   e. Proceed with caesarean section in the best interests of the baby

5. One of your colleagues has just tweeted after a long exhausting day, moaning about a complex case he had to deal with, which he believes was handed over inappropriately and mismanaged initially by another colleague. He has anonymised the case details and described the symptoms, the atypical presentation leading to initial mismanagement and the current complications making it complex.

Which one of the statements is correct with regards to maintaining confidentiality?
   a. It is acceptable to have an online conversation about the management of the complex case with your friends in the same profession
   b. It is acceptable to share your views about your colleague's clinical competencies in a closed group
   c. It is not a breach of confidentiality as the patient details are anonymised
   d. It is a breach of confidentiality as the sum of the online published information could lead to identification of the patient
   e. It is acceptable not to obtain the patient's consent for publishing this case as the details are anonymised

6. A 30-year-old para 5 woman at 36 weeks' gestation was brought in by ambulance with abdominal pain and heavy per vaginal bleeding. Her pulse was 120 bpm, blood pressure 100/60 mm Hg, respiration rate 20/min, O_2 saturation 96% on room air, and temperature 37°C. The placenta was reported as anterior high on previous scans. On examination abdomen is tender and the CTG recording is abnormal. She does not understand or speak English, but her sister who speaks English was with her. Immediate resuscitation measures were commenced and a decision for an emergency caesarean section was made by yourself.

What is the most appropriate statement in this clinical situation with regards to obtaining consent from this non-English speaker?

a. A family member is allowed to give consent on behalf of a patient for caesarean section, as she does not understand English

b. It is acceptable to obtain consent with the help of a family member or friend who speaks the same language for interpretation

c. You should obtain consent using a professional interpreter prior to the caesarean section

d. It is acceptable to use hospital employees as interpreters in day-to-day care

e. You can proceed with emergency caesarean section without consent in the best interests of the patient

Answers

1. c

EXPLANATION

A young person of any age can give valid consent to treatment as long as they are legally competent to make that decision. Usually for children under 16 years old, consent of a person with parental responsibility is required. A stepfather has no legal right to consent for the patient.

The Gillick ruling

The *Gillick* ruling in 1985 established a precedent for treating minors in the United Kingdom without their parents' consent. The ruling stated that minors of any age who are able to understand what is proposed and have 'sufficient discretion to be able to make a wise choice in their best interests' are competent to consent for medical treatment.

Persons with parental responsibility

- If the parents of a girl are not, or have not been married, only the mother automatically has legal parental responsibility.
- An unmarried father has full automatic parental responsibilities and rights over his child only where his name appears on the girl's birth certificate or the child was registered on or after 4 May 2006 (although the father may acquire the equivalent status by order or agreement or by marrying the mother of the child).
- People with parental authority (legal guardians) can consent for treatment.

Additional reading

Consent guidance on patients and doctors making decisions together. GMC website. http://www.gmc-uk.org/guidance/ethical_guidance/consent_guidance_contents.asp

StratOG.net: The Obstetrician and Gynaecologist as a professional. *Ethical and legal issues etutorial*. https://stratog.rcog.org.uk/tutorial/ethical-and-legal-issues

Treharne A, Beattie B. Consent in clinical practice. *The Obstetrician and Gynaecologist*. 2015;17:251–5. http://onlinelibrary.wiley.com/doi/10.1111/tog.12219/epdf

2. a

EXPLANATION

The Gillick ruling

The *Gillick* ruling in 1985 established a precedent for treating minors in the United Kingdom without their parents' consent. The ruling stated that minors of any age who are able to understand what is proposed and have 'sufficient discretion to be able to make a wise choice in their best interests' are competent to consent for medical treatment.

In cases of termination of pregnancy or issuing contraceptive medication for a girl under 16 years, the clinician should not contact the parents of the child unless the child agrees the clinician can do this.

Additional reading

Consent guidance on patients and doctors making decisions together. GMC website. http://www.gmc-uk.org/guidance/ethical_guidance/children_ guidance_24_26_assessing_capacity.asp

StratOG.net: The Obstetrician and Gynaecologist as a professional. *Ethical and legal issues etutorial.* https://stratog.rcog.org.uk/tutorial/ ethical-and-legal-issues

3. e

EXPLANATION

As per the Limitation Act of 1980, the limitation period (i.e. the maximum time limit within which the claimants are entitled to bring various claims) is usually 3 years from the date of the incident or date of knowledge. The date of knowledge is the date on which the claimant first had the knowledge that the injury was significant and was attributable to the act or omission alleged to constitute negligence. For children, the limitation period is 3 years from their 18th birthday. For patients with no capacity, there is no time limit.

Additional reading

StratOG.net: The Obstetrician and Gynaecologist as a professional. *Ethical and legal issues etutorial.* https://stratog.rcog.org.uk/tutorial/ ethical-and-legal-issues

4. c

EXPLANATION

Though it is a good idea to have senior help on hand, a doctor must respect the legally competent pregnant woman's right to choose or refuse any particular recommended course of action. If she makes an informed decision to refuse treatment, even when this results in her death and/or the death of her unborn child, whatever the stage of pregnancy, this decision must be respected.

It is inappropriate to invoke judicial intervention to overrule an informed and competent woman's refusal to treatment. When she has made her wishes known previously in pregnancy, even if you deem she is now legally incompetent, they must be respected.

UK law does not grant the foetus personal legal status until the time of birth (i.e. the foetus has no legal rights while it remains *in utero*).

Additional reading

Consent guidance on patients and doctors making decisions together.
GMC website. http://www.gmc-uk.org/GMC_Consent_0513_Revised. pdf_52115235.pdf
Nicholas N, El Sayed M. The changing face of consent: Past and present. *The Obstetrician and Gynaecologist*. 2006;8:39–44.
StratOG.net: The Obstetrician and Gynaecologist as a professional.
Ethical and legal issues etutorial. https://stratog.rcog.org.uk/tutorial/ethical-and-legal-issues
Treharne A, Beattie B. Consent in clinical practice. *The Obstetrician and Gynaecologist*. 2015;17:251–5. http://onlinelibrary.wiley.com/doi/10.1111/tog.12219/epdf

5. d

EXPLANATION

GMC guidance on doctors' use of social media and online behaviour – Although social media changes the means of communication, the standards expected of doctors do not change when communicating on social media rather than face to face or through other traditional media. One must be careful not to share identifiable information about patients. Although individual pieces of information may not breach confidentiality on their own, the sum of published information online could be enough to identify a patient or someone close to the patient. One must not use publicly accessible social media to discuss individual patients or their care with those patients or anyone else.

Doctors are expected to treat their colleagues fairly, with respect and to not bully, harass or make gratuitous, unsubstantiated comments about them online. The postings online are subject to the same copyright and defamation laws as written or verbal communications.

Additional reading

GMC guidance on doctors' use of social media and online behaviour. http://www.gmc-uk.org/guidance/28572.asp

6. e

EXPLANATION

If consent cannot be obtained, a clinician must act in the best interests of the patient and all decisions should be documented in the notes.

Emergency care should not be withheld or delayed because of the lack of an interpreter for non-English speakers. Professional interpreters should be available wherever possible, and use of the hospital employees is not acceptable unless in an emergency. It is unacceptable to use family or friends as interpreters, as the decision-making process can be influenced unfairly. No one can consent for a person who has capacity.

Additional reading

Consent guidance on patients and doctors making decisions together. GMC website. http://www.gmc-uk.org/GMC_Consent_0513_Revised. pdf_52115235.pdf

Treharne A, Beattie B. Consent in clinical practice. *The Obstetrician and Gynaecologist.* 2015;17:251–5. http://onlinelibrary.wiley.com/doi/10.1111/tog.12219/epdf

MEDICAL STATISTICS

Questions

1. Which one of the following statements is correct in assessing statistical correlations?
   a. Correlation coefficient tests the association between two variables
   b. It is a measure of the curvilinear association between the variables
   c. If Pearson's r is 0, there is a negative correlation
   d. Pearson's correlation depends on all the data of the observations being normal distributed
   e. A statistically significant association between two variables means it is causal

2. A correlation study shows that there is a statistically significant positive correlation between body mass index (BMI) and average blood loss at the time of caesarean section. Pearson's r is 0.4 and p value is 0.01.

   How much of the variation in blood loss can be accounted for by the BMI change?
   a. 0.16%
   b. 1.6%
   c. 0.4%
   d. 4%
   e. 16%

3. A population of pregnant women has a mean booking weight of 70 kg and the standard error of the mean is 4.

   What is the 95% confidence interval for this population?
   a. 58–82
   b. 60–80
   c. 62–78
   d. 66–74
   e. 68–72

4. In a cohort study the relationship between the use of exogenous estrogens and the risk of breast cancer was investigated in a study population of 1000 premenopausal women for a period of 8 years. The results are presented in the table.

		Breast cancer		
		Present	Absent	
Estrogen therapy	Yes	A 300	B 200	A + B = 500
	No	C 100	D 400	C + D = 500
		A + C = 400	B + D = 600	n = 1000

Which one of the following statements is correct?
a. The risk of developing breast cancer is twice more likely in the estrogen group
b. The risk of developing breast cancer is thrice more likely in the estrogen group
c. The risk of developing breast cancer is four times more likely in the estrogen group
d. The risk of developing breast cancer is five times more likely in the estrogen group
e. The risk of developing breast cancer is six times more likely in the estrogen group

5. In a cohort study, a group of 200 woman with threatened preterm labour were screened with foetal fibronectin test and the results are shown in the table.

		Preterm labour		
		Present	Absent	
Foetal Fibronectin (FFN) test	Positive	A 90	B 30	A + B = 120
	Negative	C 10	D 70	C + D = 80
		A + C = 100	B + D = 100	n = 200

Which one of the following statements is correct?
a. Sensitivity of the test is 0.9
b. Specificity of the test is 0.3
c. Positive predictive value of the test is 0.75
d. Negative predictive value of the test is 0.5
e. False-positive rate is 0.4

6. **Which one of the following statements is correct with regards to the statistical tests?**
a. Mann-Whitney compares two sets of observations on a single sample
b. Wilcoxon test compares three or more sets of observations on a single sample
c. Kruskal-Wallis test compares two independent samples drawn from the same population
d. Spearman's rank correlation coefficient assesses the strength of linear association between two variables
e. X^2 test is used for data that are not normally distributed

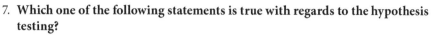

7. **Which one of the following statements is true with regards to the hypothesis testing?**
   a. Type 1 error is accepting the null hypothesis when it is false
   b. Type 2 error is rejecting the null hypothesis when it is true
   c. Alpha error is rejecting the null hypothesis when it is true
   d. Beta error is accepting the null hypothesis when it is true
   e. Gamma error is rejecting the null hypothesis when it is false

8. You are critically appraising a paper on the use of transvaginal ultrasound in diagnosing the endometrial pathology. The findings were placed in the following table.

		Hysteroscopy and endometrial biopsy	
Transvaginal ultrasound findings		Endometrial pathology present	No endometrial pathology
	Positive	A True positive 80	B False positive 10
	Negative	C False negative 20	D True negative 90
		100	100

   Which one of the statements is correct in interpreting the likelihood ratios?
   a. The positive likelihood ratio is 0.8 and is a useless test
   b. The positive likelihood ratio is 8 and is a moderately useful test
   c. The positive likelihood ratio is 8 and is a very useful test
   d. The negative likelihood ratio is 0.9 and is a very useful test
   e. The negative likelihood ratio is 0.1 and is a very useful test

Answers

1. a

The correlation coefficient or Pearson's correlation coefficient, denoted by r and the coefficient of determination, denoted by r^2 are used to measure the degree of association between two variables.

The correlation coefficient involves the use of scattergrams and is a measure of the linear association between two variables. The correlation coefficient is measured on a scale that varies from $+1$ through 0 to -1. Positive correlation between the independent and dependent variables is represented by $+1$, negative correlation by -1 and complete absence of correlation by 0.

For Pearson's correlation test, the data of at least one of the observations should be normally distributed. It should never be assumed that the statistically significant association between the two variables is causal, as it is always possible that both the variables are influenced by something else.

Additional reading

Campbell MJ, Swinscow TDV. *Statistics at Square One* (revised), Ninth edition, BMJ Publ. Group, London, 1996.

2. e

The coefficient of determination (r^2) is the square of the correlation coefficient (r). It represents the proportion of the total variation in a dependent variable that is determined by or associated with the independent variable.

In this example, $r^2 = 0.4 \times 0.4 = 0.16$. So, we can say that 16% of the variation in the average blood loss is accounted for by the BMI of the woman.

Additional reading

Campbell MJ, Swinscow TDV. *Statistics at Square One* (revised), Ninth edition, BMJ Publ. Group, London, 1996.

3. c

When the study sample comes from a larger population, the means of the different samples from the whole population will be normally distributed. The true mean of the population is not really known, but the mean of the means of the samples is the same as the population mean. The variation in the means can be described by a standard deviation, called standard error of the mean (SEM).

So, the SEM is the standard deviation of the mean of the means and it takes into account both scatter and sample size:

$$SEM = \sqrt{\frac{s^2}{n}} = \frac{s}{\sqrt{n}}$$

Confidence intervals represent the range in which 95% of the mean values would lie if the sampling was repeated under identical conditions. So, if we know the standard error, confidence intervals can be calculated using the formula **95% CI = Mean ± 1.96 × SE**.

Additional reading

Campbell MJ, Swinscow TDV. *Statistics at Square One* (revised), Ninth edition, BMJ Publ. Group, London, 1996.

4. b
Relative risk (RR) is used to compare the risk of developing a condition in two different groups of people.

RR = Probability of getting disease if exposed/probability of getting disease if not exposed.

Risk of developing breast cancer in estrogen group (event rate in the exposed group/EER) = A/A + B = 300/500 = 0.6.

Risk of developing breast cancer in control group (event rate in the control group/CER) = C/C + D = 100/500 = 0.2.

So, relative risk is (A/A + B)/(C/C + D) = 0.6/0.2 = 3.

This means that the risk of developing breast cancer is three times more likely if exposed to the exogenous estrogens than in the control group.

Additional reading

Campbell MJ, Swinscow TDV. *Statistics at Square One* (revised), Ninth edition, BMJ Publ. Group, London, 1996.

5. c
Sensitivity (true positive rate) is defined as the ability to *correctly identify individuals who have a specific disease or condition*. Sensitivity = A/A + C
Sensitivity = 90/100 = 0.9

Specificity (true negative rate) is defined as the ability to *correctly identify individuals who do not have a specific disease or condition*. Specificity = D/B + D
Specificity = 70/100 = 0.7

The false-positive rate is the proportion of false positives (B) among non-diseased (B + D), i.e. B/B + D = 0.3.

The false-negative rate is the proportion of false negatives (C) among diseased (A + C), i.e. C/A + C = 0.1.

The positive predictive value (PPV) is the proportion of true positives (A) among all positives (A + B), i.e. A/A + B.

PPV = 90/120 = 0.75

The negative predictive value (NPV) is the proportion of true negatives (D) among all negatives (C + D), i.e. D/C + D.

NPV = 70/80 = 0.875

Additional reading

Campbell MJ, Swinscow TDV. *Statistics at Square One* (revised), Ninth edition, BMJ Publ. Group, London, 1996.

6. d

All statistical tests are either parametric or non-parametric tests. Parametric tests are used when the data are normally distributed.

The following table shows some of the commonly used statistical tests.

Parametric test	Examples of equivalent non-parametric tests	Purpose of test
Two sample (unpaired) t tests	Mann-Whitney U test	Compares two independent samples drawn from the same population
One sample (paired) t test	Wilcoxon matched pairs test	Compares two sets of observations on a single sample
One-way analysis of variance (F test) using total sum of squares	Kruskal-Wallis analysis of variance by ranks	Compares three or more sets of observations on a single sample
X^2 test	Fisher's exact test	Tests the null hypothesis that the distribution of a discontinuous variable is the same in two (or more) independent samples
Product moment correlation coefficient (Pearson's r)	Spearman's rank correlation coefficient (rσ)	Assesses the strength of the straight-line association between two continuous variables
Multiple regression by least squares method	Non-parametric regression (various test)	Describes the numerical relation between a dependent variable and several predictor variables (covariates)

Additional reading

StratOG e-learning on statistical tests. https://stratog.rcog.org.uk/tutorial/research/types-of-tests-164

7. c

Truth			
		H_0 True	H_0 False
Null hypothesis decision	Accept H_0	Correct	Type 2 error
	Reject H_0	Type 1 error	Correct

Type 1 or *Alpha error* is rejecting the null hypothesis when it is true and *Type 2* or *Beta error* is accepting the null hypothesis when it is false.

Accepting a null hypothesis when it is true and rejecting a null hypothesis when it is false is correct and not an error. There is no gamma error as such.

Additional reading

Campbell MJ, Swinscow TDV. *Statistics at Square One* (revised), Ninth edition, BMJ Publ. Group, London, 1996.

StratOG e-learning on statistical tests. https://stratog.rcog.org.uk/tutorial/research/types-of-tests-164

8. b

The *likelihood ratio (LR)* represents the probability of a positive (or negative) test result in patients with disease to the probability of the same test result in patients without the disease. It indicates the ability of a test result in predicting the probability of having the event or disease and is clinically more meaningful.

Likelihood of a positive test in disease group = A/A + C = 80/100 = 0.8, and the likelihood of a positive test in a non-disease group = B/B + D = 10/100 = 0.1. So, the positive likelihood ratio is (A/A + C)/(B/B + D) = 0.8/0.1 = 8.

Similarly, the likelihood of a negative test in a disease group = C/A + C = 20/100 = 0.2, and the likelihood of a negative test in a non-disease group is D/B + D = 90/100 = 0.9. So, the negative likelihood ratio is 0.2/0.9 = 0.22.

When interpreting the likelihood ratios of a test, a positive LR of 1–5 is useless, 5–10 is moderately useful and >10 is very useful. A negative LR of 0.5–1 is useless, 0.5–0.1 is moderately useful and less than 0.1 represents a very useful test.

Additional reading

Campbell MJ, Swinscow TDV. *Statistics at Square One* (revised), Ninth edition, BMJ Publ. Group, London, 1996.

StratOG e-learning on statistical tests. https://stratog.rcog.org.uk/tutorial/research/types-of-tests-164

6 MANAGEMENT OF LABOUR AND DELIVERY

Questions

1. A 34-year-old para 2 woman with two previous normal deliveries comes in spontaneous labour at 40 weeks' gestation. She was low risk and was found to be in established labour at 6 cm cervical dilatation with intact membranes. A few hours after this examination, she had spontaneous rupture of membranes, fully dilated cervix and a brow presentation.

   What is the diameter of the presenting part?
   a. 9.5 cm
   b. 10.5 cm
   c. 11 cm
   d. 12 cm
   e. 13 cm

2. A 30-year-old para 1 woman with a previous normal vaginal delivery presents in established labour at 39 weeks' gestation. She is low risk and wants to have water birth in the midwifery-led unit. The cervix is fully effaced with 4 cm dilatation and intact membranes.

   Which one of the statements is more appropriate for care of the women labouring in water?
   a. Temperature of the water should not be more than 37°C and should be checked twice hourly
   b. Temperature of the water should not be more than 37.5°C and should be checked twice hourly
   c. Temperature of the water should not be more than 37°C and should be checked hourly
   d. Temperature of the water should not be more than 37.5°C and should be checked hourly
   e. Temperature of the water should not be more than 37°C and should be checked two hourly

3. **Which one of the following statements is correct with regards to the postures in labour?**
   a. Upright position in labour is associated with reduction in blood loss at delivery
   b. Upright position in labour has no effect on instrumental delivery rates
   c. Upright position in labour has shown a reduction in the duration of labour

d. Use of birthing balls in labour have no effect on caesarean section rates

e. Use of birthing balls in labour have been shown to reduce pain by up to 15%

4. A 35-year-old para 1 woman is in established labour with strong, regular contractions and a cervical dilatation of 4 cm. She is requesting stronger pain relief as Entonox is making her feel sick and is not very effective. She does not want an epidural and is asking about the alternative options. You have counselled her about the opioid analgesics in detail.

Which one of the following statements is true with regards to the opioid analgesics?

a. Pethidine intramuscular injection is a better analgesic than diamorphine injection

b. Diamorphine injection has shown to reduce the duration of labour

c. Remifentanil patient-controlled analgesia (PCA) is superior to epidural analgesia

d. Remifentanil PCA is contraindicated if pethidine was given previously within 6 hours

e. Remifentanil PCA needs continuous monitoring of maternal oxygen saturations

5. A 25-year-old nulliparous woman at 41 + 5 weeks' gestation was induced for postdates with Prostin followed by artificial rupture of membranes and Syntocinon infusion. She collapsed 5 minutes after epidural insertion with bradycardia and hypotension. Immediate cardiopulmonary resuscitation measures were started after stopping the epidural infusion. The collapse was believed to be secondary to inadvertent intravenous administration of the local anaesthetic causing toxicity.

What is the recommended drug of choice for the treatment of local anaesthetic toxicity?

a. Intralipid 10% intravenous bolus at 1 mL/kg over 1 minute

b. Intralipid 10% intravenous bolus at 1.5 mL/kg over 1 minute

c. Intralipid 20% intravenous bolus at 1 mL/kg over 1 minute

d. Intralipid 20% intravenous bolus at 1.5 mL/kg over 1 minute

e. Intralipid 20% intravenous bolus at 1.5 mL/kg over 2 minutes

6. A 28-year-old woman with a past history of a third-degree tear was admitted in established labour and progressed well. She was in the second stage of labour and was actively pushing with good descent.

Which one of the following would be most appropriate in preventing the obstetric anal sphincter injuries (OASIS)?

a. Cold compression during the second stage reduces the risk of OASIS

b. Mediolateral episiotomy that is 45° away from the midline when perineum is distended

c. Mediolateral episiotomy that is 60° away from the midline when perineum is distended

d. Perineal protection at crowning

e. Perineal massage throughout the antenatal period

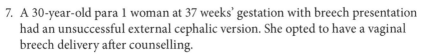

7. A 30-year-old para 1 woman at 37 weeks' gestation with breech presentation had an unsuccessful external cephalic version. She opted to have a vaginal breech delivery after counselling.

What is the risk of umbilical cord prolapse in breech presentation?
a. 1%
b. 2%
c. 3%
d. 4%
e. 5%

8. You were asked to see a para 2 woman in spontaneous labour at term who has been in the active second stage of labour for more than an hour and has maternal exhaustion. She is contracting 4–5 in 10 minutes and the cardiotocograph (CTG) is normal. Abdominal examination reveals that the head is not palpable per abdomen. She presents a fully dilated cervix, absent membranes, with a left occipitoanterior position with the vertex at +1 station.

You have decided to proceed with an operative vaginal delivery with the woman's consent. Which one of the operative vaginal deliveries would you be performing at this stage?
a. High-cavity delivery
b. Mid-cavity delivery
c. Low-cavity delivery
d. Inlet delivery
e. Outlet delivery

9. A 20-year-old nulliparous woman at 26 weeks and 4 days of gestation attends triage with a history of spotting per vaginam. On speculum examination, the cervical os was open with bulging membranes in the vagina, but there were no signs of vaginal bleeding. Your neonatal unit is full and you are arranging an *in utero* transfer.

What is the most appropriate initial management?
a. Betamethasone injection
b. Betamethasone injection and atosiban
c. Betamethasone injection and oral nifedipine
d. Betamethasone injection, atosiban and $MgSO_4$
e. Betamethasone injection, oral nifedipine and $MgSO_4$

10. A 38-year old para 1 woman at 40 weeks' gestation attends triage with a 2-hour history of spontaneous rupture of membranes (SROM). She had a previous caesarean section 3 years ago for failure to progress at 5 cm dilation and is keen to have vaginal birth after caesarean (VBAC). She is having irregular contractions, one in 10–15 minutes lasting 20 seconds. SROM was confirmed and the cervix was noted to be fully effaced and 1 cm dilated. CTG was normal at admission.

What is the most appropriate plan?
a. Await events
b. Perform continuous electronic foetal monitoring

c. Commence Syntocinon infusion

d. Reassess in 4 hours and then start Syntocinon if no progress

e. Reassess in 6 hours and then start Syntocinon if no progress

11. You were asked to see a 29-year-old nulliparous woman in the active second stage of labour, pushing for about an hour and exhausted, asking for a caesarean section. She was induced at 38 weeks for type 1 diabetes and suspected macrosomia. She is contracting 4 in 10 minutes and the CTG is normal. Per abdomen, 0/5th head was palpable and you have confirmed full dilatation, absent membranes, right occipito-posterior (ROP) position with the vertex at spines and descent to +1 during pushing.

What is the most appropriate management plan?

a. Allow another 30 minutes for pushing

b. Commence Syntocinon augmentation

c. Instrumental delivery in room

d. Trial of instrumental delivery in theatre

e. Caesarean section

12. A 36-year-old para 1 woman with a previous caesarean section for failure to progress at 7 cm was admitted at 40 + 10 weeks' gestation for induction of labour.

Which one of the statements is most appropriate with regards to her risks with induction of labour in comparison with the spontaneous VBAC labour?

a. Risk of uterine scar rupture is 1.5-fold increased

b. Risk of uterine scar rupture is two- to threefold increased

c. Risk of uterine scar rupture is fivefold increased

d. Risk of emergency caesarean section is fivefold increased

e. Risk of emergency caesarean section is two- to threefold increased

13. A nulliparous woman had a trial of instrumental delivery in theatre for failure to progress in the second stage of labour. She sustained a fourth-degree tear with 1 cm of the anal mucosa torn during the forceps delivery.

Which one of the suture materials should be used to repair the anorectal mucosa?

a. 2-0 Polyglactin (Vicryl)

b. 3-0 Polyglactin (Vicryl)

c. 2-0 Vicryl Rapide

d. 3-0 Vicryl Rapide

e. 3-0 Polydioxanone (PDS)

14. You performed forceps delivery in one of the labour ward rooms for prolonged second stage of labour and maternal exhaustion. You have diagnosed shoulder dystocia, delivered the baby in good condition with simple maneuvers. Later during the parent debriefing, you were asked about the risk of recurrence in the future.

What is her risk of shoulder dystocia in future pregnancies?

a. Same risk as the general population

b. Five times higher than the general population

c. Ten times higher than the general population

d. Fifteen times higher than the general population

e. Twenty times higher than the general population

15. You were asked by the midwife to assess the presenting part in a para 2 woman in spontaneous labour at term after SROM at 8 cm cervical dilation. She is low risk, contracting 3–4 in 10 minutes and the CTG is normal. You have confirmed that she is now fully dilated with a mento-anterior face presentation at spines.

What is the most appropriate management?

a. Caesarean section

b. Start active pushing

c. Start Syntocinon augmentation

d. Transfer to theatre for delivery

e. Allow an hour for passive second stage

16. A nulliparous woman at 40 + 2 gestation was admitted in spontaneous labour and progressed satisfactorily to full dilatation 2 hours ago. On reassessment there is no change in the descent with the vertex at −1 station, the position is occipitoanterior with absent membranes, no caput or moulding. Epidural is effective, contractions are three in 10 minutes and the CTG is normal.

What is the most appropriate management?

a. Caesarean section

b. Trial of instrumental delivery in theatre

c. Commence Syntocinon augmentation

d. Commence active second stage of labour now

e. Allow another hour for passive second stage of labour

17. A 30-year-old para 1 woman with an uncomplicated dichorionic diamniotic (DCDA) pregnancy goes into spontaneous labour at 36 weeks and delivers the first twin with cephalic presentation. The second twin is in breech presentation with good descent during contractions. The CTG is normal with four to five contractions in 10 minutes and the epidural is effective. SROM occurred with cord prolapse and the feet at the introitus.

What is the most appropriate management?

a. Transfer to theatre for caesarean section

b. Deliver by breech extraction

c. Conduct an assisted breech delivery

d. Await events for spontaneous breech delivery

e. Replace the cord and deliver breech by hands-off technique

18. You have just performed a trial of forceps in theatre and diagnosed shoulder dystocia. She has an effective epidural and had episiotomy at forceps delivery. Your team arrived for help; McRoberts manoeuvre and suprapubic pressure were not successful.

What is the most appropriate next manoeuvre in this scenario?

a. Internal manoeuvres

b. Delivery of posterior arm

c. Internal rotational manoeuvres

    d. Internal manoeuvres or all-fours position

    e. All-fours position

19. A 38-year-old, para 3 woman with gestational diabetes and pre-eclampsia was induced at 38 weeks' gestation for polyhydramnios and a big baby. She progressed well in labour and is pushing with signs of imminent delivery. She has consented for active management of the third stage of labour.

    What one of these is recommended for administration in the immediate postpartum?

    a. Syntocinon 5 IU intramuscular

    b. Syntocinon 10 IU intramuscular

    c. Syntometrine Intramuscular

    d. Ergometrine 0.5 mg intramuscular

    e. Syntocinon infusion

1. e

EXPLANATION

In brow presentation, the presenting diameter is mento-vertical, with the frontal bone as the denominator. Mento-vertical is the longest diameter at 13 cm, longer than any of the pelvic diameters. This is diagnosed when anterior fontanelle, supraorbital ridges and nose are palpable on vaginal examination.

Presentation	Presenting diameter	Diameter (cm)
Flexed vertex	Suboccipito-bregmatic	9.5
Partially deflexed vertex	Suboccipito-frontal	10.5
Deflexed vertex	Occipito-frontal	11.5
Brow	Mento-vertical	13
Face	Submento-bregmatic	9.5

Additional reading

StratOG e-learning module on Management of labour and delivery.
https://stratog.rcog.org.uk/tutorial/mechanisms-of-normal-labour-and-delivery

2. d

EXPLANATION

For women labouring in water, the temperature of the woman and the water should be checked hourly to ensure that the woman is comfortable and not becoming pyrexial. The temperature of the water should not exceed 37.5°C (National Institute for Health and Care Excellence [NICE] guidance).

Women should not enter water (a birthing pool or bath) within 2 hours of opioid administration or if they feel drowsy.

Additional reading

Alleemudder DJ et al. Analgesia for labour: An evidence-based insight for the obstetrician. *The Obstetrician and Gynaecologist*. 2015;17:147–55. http://onlinelibrary.wiley.com/doi/10.1111/tog.12196/epdf

NICE guidance CG 190 – Intrapartum care for healthy women and babies. December 2014. https://www.nice.org.uk/guidance/cg190

StratOG e-learning module on obstetric analgesia and anaesthesia. https://stratog.rcog.org.uk/tutorial/obstetric-analgesia-and-anaesthesia/analgesia-in-labour-2195

3. c

EXPLANATION

Use of a birthing ball allows a rocking movement during labour and the woman to adopt an upright position. One randomised controlled study demonstrated a 30%–40% reduction in labour pain, shorter first stage of labour, less epidural requirement and fewer caesarean sections following the implementation of a birthing ball exercise programme in labour.

A Cochrane systematic review ($n = 5218$) supported adopting an upright position during labour and has shown a reduction in analgesic requirements, shorter first stage of labour of 1 hour 20 minutes, shorter second stage of labour, reduction in caesarean sections, instrumental delivery rates and episiotomies, but it has also shown an increase in blood loss.

Additional reading

Alleemudder DJ et al. Analgesia for labour: An evidence-based insight for the obstetrician. *The Obstetrician and Gynaecologist*. 2015;17:147–55. http://onlinelibrary.wiley.com/doi/10.1111/tog.12196/epdf

StratOG e-learning module on obstetric analgesia and anaesthesia. https://stratog.rcog.org.uk/tutorial/obstetric-analgesia-and-anaesthesia/analgesia-in-labour-2195

4. e

EXPLANATION

A two-centre double-blind randomised controlled trial ($n = 406$ women) has compared the analgesic efficacy of intramuscular pethidine and intramuscular diamorphine (IDvIP trial) and the results have shown that intramuscular 7.5 mg diamorphine is a significantly better analgesic than 150 mg pethidine injection. Diamorphine injection has prolonged delivery by 82 minutes, but there were no significant differences in neonatal adverse outcomes with either analgesic.

Remifentanil PCA is an ultrafast-acting opioid that takes 5 minutes to work and provides pain relief on demand when given via a PCA pump. Its use is contraindicated if morphine or pethidine were given in the previous 4 hours. Continuous monitoring of maternal oxygen saturation is mandatory during its use due to its association with respiratory depression and cardiorespiratory arrest (<1 in 2200).

A meta-analysis of five studies comparing epidural with remifentanil PCA has shown that remifentanil is not superior to epidural in analgesic efficacy.

Additional reading

Alleemudder DJ et al. Analgesia for labour: An evidence-based insight for the obstetrician. *The Obstetrician and Gynaecologist*. 2015;17:147–55. http://onlinelibrary.wiley.com/doi/10.1111/tog.12196/epdf

StratOG e-learning module on obstetric analgesia and anaesthesia. https://stratog.rcog.org.uk/tutorial/obstetric-analgesia-and-anaesthesia/analgesia-in-labour-2195

5. d

EXPLANATION

Cardiopulmonary resuscitation should be continued throughout treatment with lipid emulsion. Recovery from local anaesthetic–induced cardiac arrest may take more than an hour. Propofol is not a suitable substitute for lipid emulsion, and lignocaine should not be used as an anti-arrhythmic therapy.

An intravenous bolus injection of 20% lipid emulsion (Intralipid is the most commonly used brand name) at 1.5 mL/kg should be given over a minute followed by an intravenous infusion of 20% lipid emulsion at 15 mL/kg/h.

If cardiovascular stability has not been restored or there is deterioration of adequate circulation, repeat two more boluses of intravenous 20% lipid emulsion 5 minutes apart (maximum of three boluses including the first one). Intravenous infusion can be doubled at 30 mL/kg/h after 5 minutes of bolus if cardiovascular stability has not been restored or deterioration of adequate circulation occurs. Infusion can be continued until stable or maximum dose of lipid emulsion was given.

Additional reading

Management of severe local anaesthetic toxicity. The association of anaesthetists of Great Britain and Ireland (AAGBI) guidance. https://www.aagbi.org/sites/default/files/la_toxicity_2010_0.pdf

StratOG e-learning module on obstetric analgesia and anaesthesia. https://stratog.rcog.org.uk/tutorial/obstetric-analgesia-and-anaesthesia/analgesia-in-labour-2195

6. d

EXPLANATION

Clinicians should explain to women that the evidence for the protective effect of episiotomy is conflicting. Mediolateral episiotomy should be considered in instrumental deliveries and where episiotomy is indicated, the mediolateral technique is recommended, with careful attention to ensure that the angle is 60° away from the midline when the perineum is distended. There is no indication for episiotomy in this clinical scenario.

Perineal protection at crowning can be protective. Warm compression during the second stage of labour reduces the risk of OASIS. No differences were seen in the incidence of first- or second-degree perineal tears or third- or fourth-degree perineal trauma with the perineal massage.

Additional reading

The management of third- and fourth-degree perineal tears. *Green-top guideline No 29*. June 2015. https://www.rcog.org.uk/globalassets/documents/guidelines/gtg-29.pdf

7. a

EXPLANATION

The overall incidence of umbilical cord prolapse ranges from 0.1% to 0.6%. In the case of breech presentation, the incidence is higher at 1%.

Additional reading

Umbilical cord prolapse. Green-top guideline No 50. https://www.rcog.org.uk/globalassets/documents/guidelines/gtg-50-umbilicalcordprolapse-2014.pdf

8. b

EXPLANATION

Operative vaginal delivery classification is as follows:

Outlet delivery is when the foetal skull has reached the pelvic floor with the foetal head at or on the perineum and the foetal scalp is visible without parting the labia. Sagittal suture is in the anterior-posterior diameter or right or left occiput anterior or posterior position (rotation does not exceed 45°).

Low-cavity delivery is when the leading point of the foetal skull is at or lower than the +2 station, but not on the pelvic floor.

Mid-cavity delivery is when the leading point of the foetal skull is between the ischial spines and +2 station with either one-fifth or less head palpable per abdomen.

High-cavity delivery is when the leading point of the foetal skull is above the ischial spines with more than two-fifths head palpable per abdomen. Vaginal operative delivery is not indicated as the presenting part is at this level.

Additional reading

Available at: https://www.rcog.org.uk/globalassets/documents/guidelines/gtg_26.pdf

9. c

EXPLANATION

As this patient has a high possibility of preterm labour at 26 + 4 weeks' gestation, maternal corticosteroids should be offered. Oral nifedipine is the first line for tocolysis to women in suspected or diagnosed preterm labour between 26 + 0 and 33 + 6 weeks of pregnancy with intact membranes, and it should be offered. If nifedipine is contraindicated, offer oxytocin receptor antagonists for tocolysis.

Intravenous magnesium sulfate ($MgSO_4$) for neuroprotection of the baby should be offered if women are in established preterm labour or are having a planned preterm birth within 24 hours between 24 + 0 and 29 + 6 weeks of pregnancy and should be considered for women between 30 + 0 and 33 + 6 weeks of pregnancy.

Additional reading

Preterm labour and birth – NICE guideline 25, November 2015. https://www.nice. org.uk/guidance/ng25

10. a

EXPLANATION

As this woman is not in established labour with no regular contractions and the admission CTG is normal, there is no need for continuous electronic foetal monitoring.

Women should be advised to have continuous electronic foetal monitoring for the duration of planned VBAC, commencing at the onset of regular uterine contractions. There should be continuous monitoring of the labour to ensure prompt identification of maternal or foetal compromise, labour dystocia or uterine scar rupture. Consequently, all women in established VBAC labour should receive: supportive one-to-one care, intravenous access with full blood count and blood group and save, continuous electronic foetal monitoring, regular monitoring of maternal symptoms and signs and regular (no less than 4-hourly) assessment of their progress in labour.

Additional reading

Birth after previous caesarean birth. *Green-top guideline No 45.* October 2015. https://www.rcog.org.uk/globalassets/documents/guidelines/gtg_45.pdf

11. d

EXPLANATION

Operative vaginal births that have a higher risk of failure should be considered for a trial and conducted in a place where immediate recourse to caesarean section can be undertaken. Higher rates of failure are associated with

- Maternal body mass index (BMI) over 30
- Estimated foetal weight over 4000 g or clinically big baby
- Occipito-posterior position
- Mid-cavity delivery or when one-fifth of the head palpable per abdomen

Trial of instrumental delivery in theatres is the most appropriate plan in this case as the mother is exhausted, with ROP at spines, that is, mid-cavity instrumental delivery of a suspected big baby.

Additional reading

Operative vaginal delivery. Green-top guideline No 26. 2011. https://www.rcog.org.uk/globalassets/documents/guidelines/gtg_26.pdf

12. b

EXPLANATION

Women should be informed of the two- to threefold increased risk of uterine rupture and around 1.5-fold increased risk of caesarean delivery in induced and/or augmented labour compared with spontaneous VBAC labour.

Clinicians should be aware that induction of labour using mechanical methods (amniotomy or Foley catheter) is associated with a lower risk of scar rupture compared with induction using prostaglandins.

Additional reading

Birth after previous caesarean birth. *Green-top guideline No 45*. October 2015. https://www.rcog.org.uk/globalassets/documents/guidelines/gtg_45.pdf

13. b

EXPLANATION

3-0 Polyglactin should be used to repair the anorectal mucosa as it may cause less irritation and discomfort than polydioxanone (PDS) sutures. The torn anorectal mucosa should be repaired with sutures using either the continuous or interrupted technique.

Additional reading

The management of third- and fourth-degree perineal tears. *Green-top guideline No 29*. 2015. https://www.rcog.org.uk/globalassets/documents/guidelines/gtg-29.pdf

14. c

EXPLANATION

The rate of shoulder dystocia in women who have had a previous shoulder dystocia has been reported to be 10 times higher than the rate in the general population.

Additional reading

Shoulder dystocia. *COG Green-top guideline No 42*. 2012. https://www.rcog.org.uk/globalassets/documents/guidelines/gtg_42.pdf

15. e

EXPLANATION

It is possible for the mento-anterior face presentation to have a normal vaginal delivery. As the labour progress is good, there is no need to intervene, and this presentation itself is not an indication per se for delivery in theatre. Hence, allow an hour for the passive descent of the presenting part. Caesarean section is recommended for the mento-posterior face presentation.

Additional reading

RCOG e-learning: stratog.rcog.org.uk: Management of labour and delivery. https://stratog.rcog.org.uk/tutorial/easi-resource/direct-op-and-face-deliveries-5137

16. c

EXPLANATION

As there is no progress/change in the descent of the presenting part during the last 2 hours, starting Syntocinon augmentation is the most appropriate option. Oxytocin is advised if contractions are inadequate or if there is a delay secondary to malposition or if there is little or no descent of the head.

As the CTG is normal, there is no indication for immediate delivery with either instrumental delivery or caesarean section.

Additional reading

NICE Guideline [CG190]: Intrapartum care for healthy women and babies. 2014. https://www.nice.org.uk/guidance/cg190
RCOG e-learning: Management of labour and delivery. https://stratog.rcog.org.uk/tutorial/assessment-of-progress-in-labour/delay-in-labour-2045

17. b

EXPLANATION

Deliver by breech extraction is most appropriate in this case as delivery needs to be expedited due to the presence of cord prolapse. Favourable factors for preterm vaginal breech delivery include para 1, uncomplicated DCDA twin pregnancy, vaginal delivery of twin a few minutes ago, good contractions and effective analgesia.

Additional reading

RCOG e-learning: Intrapartum management of multiple pregnancy. https://stratog.
rcog.org.uk/tutorial/intrapartum-management-of-multiple-pregnancy

18. a

EXPLANATION

Internal manoeuvres or 'all-fours' position should be used if McRoberts
manoeuvre and suprapubic pressure fail. As the epidural is effective in this case,
internal manoeuvres would be more appropriate than the all-fours position. Either
the delivery of the posterior arm or internal rotational manoeuvres can be tried
first depending on the clinical circumstances and operator experience.

Additional reading

Shoulder dystocia. Green-top guideline No 42. 2012. https://www.rcog.org.uk/
globalassets/documents/guidelines/gtg_42.pdf

19. b

EXPLANATION

NICE guidance: For active management of third stage, administer 10 IU of
oxytocin by intramuscular injection with the birth of the anterior shoulder
or immediately after the birth of the baby and before the cord is clamped and
cut. Oxytocin use is advised as it is associated with fewer side effects than the
syntometrine.

In this scenario, syntometrine and ergometrine usage is contraindicated due to
the history of pre-eclampsia.

Additional reading

NICE Guideline [CG190]: Intrapartum care for healthy women and babies. 2014.
https://www.nice.org.uk/guidance/cg190

GYNAECOLOGICAL ONCOLOGY

Questions

1. A 60-year-old woman is referred to the rapid access 2 week wait clinic with vulval itching and soreness. Vulval examination reveals small ivory-coloured slightly raised areas which join to form white patches in a figure-of-eight distribution. Vaginal introitus is narrowed with atrophy of the labia minora. Vulval mapping biopsies reveal lichen sclerosus.

   Her associated risks include all of the following except which one condition?
   a. Increased risk of a personal history of autoimmune disorders
   b. Increased risk of a family history of autoimmune disorders
   c. An associated thyroid disorder
   d. An associated pernicious anaemia
   e. Vesiculobullous autoimmune disease of anogenital site

2. A 40-year-old woman presents with severe vulval pruritus. Vulvoscopy reveals acetowhite areas following application of acetic acid. Vulval mapping biopsy reveals usual type (human papilloma virus [HPV] related) of VIN.

   She can be treated with which one of the following methods?
   a. Radical vulvectomy
   b. Simple vulvectomy
   c. Therapeutic human papilloma virus vaccine
   d. Interferon therapy
   e. Local surgical excision

3. A 24-year-old woman presents to her GP with abdominal pain. Clinical examination reveals a large abdomino-pelvic mass. She is referred to a rapid access 2-week wait clinic. Following investigations, computed tomography (CT) scan reveals left-sided solid ovarian mass with raised serum lactate dehydrogenase (LDH) enzyme levels. She undergoes fertility sparing surgery and the histology reveals nests of tumour cells (vesicular cells with clear cytoplasm and central nuclei) separated by fibrous stroma infiltrated with T lymphocytes.

   Which is the most likely type of ovarian tumour in her case?
   a. Brenner tumour
   b. Immature teratoma

c. Endodermal sinus tumour

    d. Dysgerminoma

    e. Embryonal carcinoma

4. A 48-year-old is referred to rapid access clinic with postmenopausal bleeding. Her ultrasound shows endometrial thickness of 5.1 mm. She gives family history of endometrial cancer in the mother (died at the age of 44 years), her brother died of bowel cancer at the age of 44 years and her sister died of ovarian cancer at the age of 46 years. She is anxious that she has a genetic history and worried that she has inherited some genetic condition.

   The patient is at increased risk of which one of the following?

    a. Breast cancer

    b. Bowel cancer

    c. Cervical cancer

    d. Endometrial cancer

    e. Ovarian cancer

5. A 70-year-old woman is referred to rapid access clinic. Her main symptom is vulval itching and soreness. Vulval examination reveals erythematous vulva with excoriation and lichenification. Vulval biopsy shows large pleomorphic cells with amphophilic, granular cytoplasm and prominent nucleus and mainly located in the lower portion of the epidermis. Occasional signet cells were seen. The cells stained positive with mucicarmine and PAS. Immunohistochemical studies showed positivity with EMA, CAM 5.2, CK7 and GCDFP-15. The doctor recommends vulval excision.

   What is the most likely diagnosis in her case?

    a. Plasma cell vulvitis

    b. Vulval Crohn disease

    c. Malignant melanoma

    d. Bowen disease

    e. Extramammary Paget disease

6. A 30-year-old woman with a normal smear 3 years ago has a current smear reported as mild dyskaryosis. A high-risk HPV test on the liquid-based cytology (LBC) sample is positive. She is referred to colposcopy clinic. Colposcopy reveals CIN2 and therefore a large loop excision of transformation zone (LLETZ) is performed.

   The next management step in her case is which one of the following?

    a. HPV testing in 6 months

    b. Cytology follow-up at 12 months with colposcopy

    c. Cytology follow-up at 6 months

    d. Cytology follow-up at 6 months with HPV testing

    e. Cytology follow-up at 12 months with HPV testing

7. A 40-year-old woman para 2 presents with bloating and abdominal swelling. Her mother died of ovarian cancer and her sister died of breast cancer at the ages of 50 and 40, respectively. A genetic screening test reveals that she is carrier of *BRCA1* gene.

Her management include the following except for which of the following?

a. Risk-reducing bilateral salpingo-oophorectomy (RRBSO)
b. Risk-reducing breast surgery (bilateral mastectomy)
c. Screening for ovarian cancer
d. Breast screening
e. Counselling regarding 1%–6% risk of primary peritoneal cancer even after oophorectomy

8. A 45-year-old woman presents to GP with abdominal bloating. A blood test was performed for Ca125 which measures 1000 units/mL. She is referred to rapid access clinic (gynaecological oncology). A CT scan (chest, abdomen and pelvis) reveals a large abdominal mass possibly filled with mucin. The findings are suggestive of mucinous carcinoma. She undergoes staging laparotomy which reveals pre-operative rupture of the cyst with ascites and mucinous substance filling the abdomen. The histology is reported as mucinous carcinoma of the left ovary with rupture of cyst.

What is the International Federation of Gynecology and Obstetrics (FIGO) stage in her case?

a. IB
b. IC1
c. IC2
d. IC3
e. IIA

9. A 62-year-old woman is referred to rapid access clinic (gynaecological oncology) for postmenopausal bleeding (PMB). An ultrasound scan reveals thickened endometrium. Hysteroscopy and endometrial biopsy show Grade 1 endometrial cancer. A magnetic resonance imaging (MRI) scan was performed for staging which reveals cervical involvement. She undergoes total abdominal hysterectomy and bilateral salpingo-oophorectomy (TAH+BSO). The final histology reveals Grade 1 endometrioid carcinoma with less than half myometrial invasion and involvement of cervical glands.

What is the FIGO stage in her case?

a. IA
b. IB
c. II
d. IIIA
e. IIIB

10. A 55-year-old woman is referred to rapid access clinic (gynaecological oncology) for PMB. An ultrasound scan reveals thickened endometrium and a solid ovarian mass on the left side. An endometrial Pipelle biopsy shows grade 1 endometrioid carcinoma. She undergoes TAH+BSO. Her Ca125 (150 units/mL) and inhibin B levels (100 ng/L) are elevated. She undergoes staging laparotomy (TAH+BSO, omentectomy, peritoneal biopsies and peritoneal washings and look around inside the abdomen).

What would be the likely histological diagnosis of ovarian mass in her case?
a. Polyembryoma
b. Granulose cell tumour
c. Sertoli-stromal cell tumour
d. Gynandroblastoma
e. Serous cystadenocarcinoma

11. A 20-year-old woman presents to GP with abdominal distension. She is referred to rapid access clinic (gynaecological oncology). Her Ca125 is 100, CEA, AFP, ß-HCG, LDH are normal. CT scan reveals a large solid mass arising from the left ovary with normal right ovary. She undergoes staging laparotomy with fertility preservation. The histology reveals immature grade 2 neural tissue.

    What is the histological diagnosis in this case?
    a. Struma ovarii
    b. Mature teratoma
    c. Glioblastoma
    d. Neuroblastoma
    e. Immature teratoma

12. **A patient is noted to have symmetrical bilateral ovarian tumours which are removed. The histopathology report reveals tumour cells show signet ring morphology and raise the possibility that these represent metastasis rather than primary ovarian malignancy. Which is the most likely primary site?**
    a. Cervix
    b. Thymus
    c. Pancreas
    d. Stomach
    e. Thyroid

13. A 74-year-old woman presents to rapid access clinic with vulval soreness. Examination reveals a 2 cm mass on the right labia away from the midline. A biopsy of the lesion from the margin of the tumour reveals squamous cell carcinoma with depth of invasion <1 mm. The MRI of the pelvis reveals the same vulva mass with no other abnormality. Her case is subsequently discussed in the multidisciplinary team meeting.

    The management of this patient involves which one of the following?
    a. Radical vulvectomy
    b. Radical vulvectomy with bilateral groin lymphadenectomy
    c. Radical vulvectomy with groin lymphadenectomy on the same side
    d. Wide local excision of vulval lesion
    e. Wide local excision of vulval lesion with groin lymphadenectomy on the same side

14. A 25-year-old woman is 14 weeks' pregnant. She has a moderate dyskaryosis in the cervical smear and is referred to the colposcopic clinic.

    How would you manage her?
    a. Colposcopy and LLETZ
    b. Colposcopy to rule out invasive disease and follow-up in colposcopy clinic at 3 months post-delivery

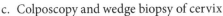

   c. Colposcopy and wedge biopsy of cervix
   d. No need for colposcopy during pregnancy as it is difficult to interpret findings on cervix
   e. Discharge the patient to GP if colposcopy is normal

15. A 62-year-old woman presents with one episode of postmenopausal bleeding. Ultrasound scan shows endometrial thickness (ET) of 4 mm and bilateral ovarian cyst 7 × 8 × 9 cm each. They are multilocular and partly solid, partly cystic with thick walls. CA-125 is 30.

    What is the recommended management in her case?
    a. Manage locally in gynaecological oncology unit with laparotomy and oophorectomy
    b. Manage locally in gynaecological oncology unit with laparotomy and pelvic clearance
    c. Refer her to cancer centre for further management
    d. Conservative treatment
    e. Manage in gynaecological oncology centre with laparoscopic oophorectomy

16. A 26-year-old woman is referred to colposcopy clinic for severe dyskaryosis. Colposcopy reveals a tumour on the cervix. Cervical biopsy is reported as squamous cell carcinoma of cervix. She has been booked for radical hysterectomy.

    Which of these instruments is used to identify and release the ureter in the ureteric tunnel in radical hysterectomy?
    a. Gullums
    b. Zaplins
    c. Rogers
    d. Roberts
    e. Lahey

17. A 28-year-old woman is referred for colposcopy with abnormal smear reported as severe dyskaryosis. Colposcopy reveals a high-grade lesion. She subsequently undergoes LLETZ procedure under general anaesthesia in view of anxiety. The final histology reveals cervical cancer (microinvasion <3 mm depth of invasion and horizontal spread of <7 mm). The margins of LLETZ reveal cervical intra-epithelial neoplasia 3 (CIN3).

    What should be her subsequent management?
    a. Follow-up for colposcopy and smear with HPV testing
    b. Repeat LLETZ
    c. Radical hysterectomy
    d. Simple hysterectomy
    e. Laparoscopic pelvic lymphadenectomy

Answers

1. e

LICHEN SCLEROSUS (LS)

It is a relatively uncommon condition (between 1 in 70 and 1 in 1000 women) which can occur at any age (it can even occur prior to puberty) but is more common in postmenopausal women (1 in 30 women). Although it can occur anywhere, it is more common in the genital areas (vulva is most common site in women). Higgins and Cruickshank indicated that at least 25% of women seen in dedicated vulva clinics received treatment for vulval LS. Evidence suggests that it is an autoimmune condition, with around 40% of women either having or developing other autoimmune conditions (circulating auto-antibodies are more common in women with lichen planus than with LS). The common conditions associated with LS include thyroid disorders, alopecia areata, pernicious anaemia and type 1 diabetes mellitus. The reported prevalence of autoimmune conditions in first-degree relatives is around 30%. Involvement of anogenital sites with vesiculobullous autoimmune diseases is uncommon.

Symptoms

The most common symptom is vulval itching which may worse at night (itching is related to active inflammation with erythema and keratinisation of vulval skin). White patches with areas of wrinkled tissue paper can be seen on parts of the vulva (this is described as lichenification). These areas are fragile and easily bruise with scratching and give rise to splitting of the skin. The inner labia and introitus may shrink leading to introital narrowing causing vulval soreness and painful sexual intercourse. Often the skin is atrophic and continuing inflammation results in adhesions (causes fusion of labia minora and lateral margins of the clitoris). Occasionally the vaginal opening is closed with fusion of labia minora and can cause difficulty with micturition (spraying of urine) and or urinary retention.

Diagnosis

The diagnosis is made based on clinical examination. The indications for vulval mapping biopsies include failure to respond to treatment, clinical suspicion of vulval intraepithelial neoplasia (VIN) or cancer, or if there is clinical uncertainty.

Risks

There is increased risk of VIN developing in LS, and this is usually differentiated-type VIN. A differentiated type of VIN may need skinning vulvectomy as it is likely to progress into cancer.

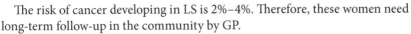

The risk of cancer developing in LS is 2%–4%. Therefore, these women need long-term follow-up in the community by GP.

The other risks or complications of LS include

- Development of clitoral pseudo-cyst
- Sexual dysfunction
- Dysaesthesia
- Labial fusion

Treatment

Management is usually by ultrapotent topical steroids.

Clobetasol Propionate 0.05%

The highest response rates are seen with longer regular use before returning to as required use and also in women under 50 years of age. It appears to be safe and effective in premenarchal girls. The relapse rate is 84% within 4 years.

The steroid cream needs to be applied sparingly to the areas of itch or discomfort or changes on the skin.

Once daily for 1 month
Then alternate days for 1 month
Then twice weekly for 1 month
Then once a week for 1 month

Then gradually reduce the frequency until you can use it occasionally or stop. (This regimen may need to be varied depending on response rate.) All patients need a long-term moisturiser to be used at least twice a day.

Note: The British Association of Dermatologists is about to publish a new guideline on this.

In 4%–10% of women with anogenital LS, symptoms will not improve with the above steroids (steroid-resistant disease) and may need second-line treatment in the form of topical tacrolimus. Such treatments need supervision in a specialist clinic.

Additional reading

Higgins CA, Cruickshank ME. A population-based case-control study of aetiological factors associated with vulval lichen sclerosus. *Journal of Obstetrics and Gynaecology.* 2012;32(3):271–5. http://www.medscape.com/viewarticle/820436_2

Management of vulval skin disorders. *Green-top guideline No 58.* February 2011. https://www.rcog.org.uk/en/guidelines-research-services/guidelines/gtg58/

UK National Guideline on the Management of Vulval Conditions. Clinical Effectiveness Group, British Association for Sexual Health and HIV. February 2014. http://www.bashh.org/documents/UK%20national%20guideline%20for%20the%20management%20of%20vulval%20conditions%202014.pdf

2. e

VULVAL INTRAEPITHELIAL NEOPLASIA (VIN)

It is a precancerous condition of the vulval region. It is classified into two types: (1) usual type which is associated with HPV or (2) differentiated type which occurs in the background of LS. Both types of VIN can progress to develop into cancer (the risk of progression is 40%–60%) and is higher in untreated women.

Differences between usual type and differentiated type of VIN

Differentiated type VIN	Classic or usual type of VIN
Rarer than usual type of VIN.	Most common type of VIN.
More common in their 60s–80s.	More common in women in their 30s–50s.
Not related to HPV infection.	HPV related (especially HPV 16).
Commonly associated with LS and may be associated with lichen planus.	Associated with Bowen disease.
Both VIN and LS or lichen planus seen next to each other on examination; linked to keratinising squamous cell carcinoma.	Classified into warty, basaloid and mixed pathological subtypes.
Usually unifocal disease.	Usually associated with multifocal disease (i.e. cervical intraepithelial neoplasia [CIN], vaginal intraepithelial neoplasia [VAIN], anal intraepithelial neoplasia [AIN]).
Malignant potential is high.	Other risk factors include smoking, sexual promiscuity and chronic immunosuppression.
Treatment involves local surgical excision. Emollient and mild steroid may help to relieve symptoms of pruritus. Therapies such as antiviral and vaccination are unlikely to be successful treatment or preventive strategies.	Treatment involves local surgical excision. The risk of recurrence with excision is same as vulvectomy. The risk of recurrence is reduced if the margins are clear. Topical imiquimod, an immune-response modifier and laser ablation are effective methods of treatment for genital warts and VIN.

Surgical treatment

The indications for treatment include symptom relief, rule invasive disease and reduce the risk of developing invasive cancer (12%–17% undergoing excision of VIN have unrecognised invasive disease).

The standard treatment of VIN is local surgical excision. Simple or radical vulvectomy is not appropriate in view of adverse effects on body image and sexual function. The recurrence rate with local excision is the same as vulvectomy. The risk of recurrence is reduced if the margins are clear of disease. Complete response rates are higher with excision than with ablative therapy or medical treatments. Reconstructive vulval surgery can be offered to these women especially if a wider area needs to be excised, and this has shown good sexual function in small case series.

Non-surgical treatments

Medical treatments can be used as alternatives to surgery but would need good compliance of patients (as need regular and long-term follow-up). These treatments preserve anatomy of the vulva and avoid surgical complications.

Agents used to treat VIN

Topical imiquimod cream (licensed for used in genital warts) has been used to treat VIN with 15%–81% clinical and histological response rates. The side effects include erythema, pain and swelling and can lead to non-compliance (if these patients do not finish the 16-week course of treatment).

Cidofovir is also used to treat genital warts and has shown some clinical and histological responses in VIN. Trial results are awaited for its place in treatment.

Long-term outcomes and risk of invasion are not known with the above medical treatments.

Laser ablation

Laser ablation has been shown to be effective in small case studies. However it cannot be used in hair bearing skin owing to involvement of skin appendages and also treatment failure rates are high (40%). It is useful when glans and hood of clitoris need preservation or when surgery is contraindicated.

Other treatments

There is currently insufficient evidence to suggest the use of Cavitron ultrasonic surgical aspiration, photodynamic therapy, interferons and therapeutic HPV vaccine.

Follow-up

Regular follow-up (at least annual follow-up) with clinical assessment and vulvoscopy is required in these women. Even after surgical excision, 4% of these women have a residual risk of developing cancer. These women are also at risk of developing intraepithelial neoplasia (precancerous disease) at other lower genital tract (this is called field phenomenon) sites (cervix, vagina and perianal region). Therefore, colposcopy of these sites is important at follow-up, especially if the VIN is the usual type. (This is usually multicentre disease.) Many of these women are smokers, and they should be strongly advised to stop smoking and given help where appropriate.

Additional reading

BASHH. 2014 UK National Guideline on the Management of Vulval Conditions. Clinical Effectiveness Group, British Association for Sexual Health and HIV. February 2014. https://www.bashh.org/documents/UK%20national%20 guideline%20for%20the%20management%20of%20vulval%20conditions%20 2014.pdf
Management of vulval skin disorders. Green-top guideline No 58. February 2011.

3. d

GERM CELL TUMOURS

Germ cell tumours account for 10% of all ovarian tumours. They are derived from the primitive germ cells of embryonic gonad and usually occur in young women in their 20s. The major issue in managing these women is to be able to preserve fertility and at the same time not compromise the chances of cure.

Germ cell tumours may produce tumour markers specific to their cell type. These include the following:

- α-Fetoprotein (AFP): endodermal sinus tumour
- AFP and βHCG: Embryonal carcinoma (also can produce oestradiol)
- βHCG: Non-gestational choriocarcinoma
- βHCG: Gestational trophoblastic disease
- βHCG may be raised: Dysgerminoma (3% of cases)
- Placental alkaline phosphatase and LDH: Dysgerminoma (especially metastatic disease)

Dysgerminoma (equivalent of seminomas in males) is the most common type of germ cell tumour and commonly occurs in adolescents and women of reproductive age. Sixty percent of these cases are diagnosed in women younger than 20 years of age. The clinical signs and symptoms can include any one of the following; abdominal pain, abdominal mass, fever and rarely ascites.

Dysgerminomas are bilateral in 10% of the cases. They are composed of germ cells that have not differentiated to form embryonic or extra-embryonic structures. The tumour cells very much resemble primordial germ cells and normally do not secrete hormones. However, raised βHCG is seen in 3% of these tumours and a small percentage may secrete α-fetoprotein. Serum LDH and placental alkaline phosphatase may be raised. Rarely, it can be associated with hypercalcaemia. In young women with primary amenorrhoea and gonadal dysgenesis, it can be associated with gonadoblastoma. Histologically, lymphocytic infiltration in the stroma is hallmark of these tumours.

The primary treatment is surgery followed by adjuvant chemotherapy in cases more than stage IA. They are highly sensitive to radiotherapy but the associated complications (secondary leukaemia and infertility) prohibit its use. The overall prognosis is good and 5-year survival is 90%. Metastatic spread often involves retroperitoneal and pelvic lymph nodes. Distant metastasis to lung, bone and liver has been reported via haematogenous spread.

Additional reading

Kumar B, Davies-Humphreys J. Tumour markers and ovarian cancer screening. Personal assessment in continuing education. *Reviews, Questions and Answers*. RCOG press. February 2003;3:51–3.

Sanusi FA, Carter P, Barton DPJ. Non epithelial ovarian cancers. Personal assessment in continuing education. *Reviews, Questions and Answers*. RCOG press. February 2003;3:38–9.

4. d

HEREDITARY NONPOLYPOSIS COLORECTAL CANCER (HNPCC)

This woman is likely to have Lynch syndrome (HNPCC) which is an autosomal dominant condition. (This means that people with HNPCC have a 50% chance of passing the gene mutation to each of their children.) The vast majority of individuals with HNPCC will develop cancer. The hallmark of this condition is DNA mismatch repair defect. (These genes are called *MLH1*, *MSH2*, *MSH6* and *PMS2*.)

The predisposition to cancer is usually in the third and fourth decades of life although it can occur at other ages. These women are at high risk of developing early onset of multiple types of cancer including colorectal (most common and accounts for 2%–5% of colon cancers), endometrium (second most common cancer), ovarian, gastric, small bowel, upper urinary tract (ureteric and renal pelvic cancers), brain (most common type; glioblastoma), small intestine and hepatobiliary tract.

The lifetime risk of colon, endometrial and ovarian cancers in women who carry this gene are 50%–80%, 40%–60% and 10%–12% respectively. The risk of endometrial cancer in the general population is 3%. If the woman is carrying *MSH6* mutation (Lynch syndrome), the risk of endometrial cancer may exceed the risk of colorectal cancer. The risk of ovarian cancer in the general population is 1.4%.

Unlike *BRCA*-related ovarian cancers, which are usually high-grade serous tumour, Lynch syndrome–associated ovarian carcinomas are often early stage and moderately or well differentiated. Synchronous endometrial and ovarian cancers are common in women with Lynch syndrome.

Additional reading

Management of women with genetic predisposition to gynaecological cancers. RCOG: Scientific impact paper No 48. February 2015. http://gut.bmj.com/content/early/2013/02/20/gutjnl-2012-304356.long

Revised guidelines for the clinical management of Lynch syndrome (HNPCC): Recommendations by a group of European experts. http://www.ouh.nhs.uk/patient-guide/leaflets/files%5C10055Plynchsyndrome.pdf

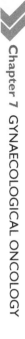

5. e

OTHER VULVAL CONDITIONS

Vulval condition	Extramammary paget	Plasma cell vulvitis	Vulval psoriasis	Vulval candidiasis	Behçet disease	Crohn disease
Frequency	Rare	Rare, aetiology unknown; also named as Zoon vulvitis	Rare	Uncommon	Rare	Rare
Association	Usually associated with underlying adenocarcinoma	Chronic inflammatory condition	Mainly involves vulval skin but not vaginal epithelium	Vagina and vulva are common sites; may involve other systems	Chronic multisystem disease	Chronic inflammatory bowel disease
Age	Common in postmenopausal women	Common in postmenopausal women		Common with steroid and antibiotic use, obesity, diabetes mellitus and immunosuppression		Common in women with history of Crohn disease
Symptoms	Presents with vulval pruritus and soreness	Presents with vulval pruritus, burning dyspareunia and dysuria	Vulval irritation	Presents with vulval irritation, itching and soreness	Presents with recurrent oral and genital ulcers (can involve the cervix, vulva and vagina)	Presents with vulval swelling, ulceration or sinus formation
Histology/ physical morphology	Large pleomorphic cells (lower portion of the epidermis); treatment is surgical excision	Histology: plasma cell dermal infiltration, vessel dilatation, haemosiderin deposition	Vulva: smooth, non-scaly red or pink discrete lesions	Chronic vulval inflammation that extends from inner labia to medial part of thighs and mons pubis	Ulcers usually recurrent and painful and heal with scarring	Vulva is swollen and oedematous with granulomas or draining sinuses or ulceration
Treatment	Surgical margins are difficult to achieve; recurrence is common; limited success with photodynamic therapy and topical imiquimod	Limited evidence: may benefit from topical ultrapotent steroids and emollients	Emollients, soap substitutes, topical steroids and calcipotriene are used for symptom control	Oral and topical antifungal therapy; may need combination with a steroid cream if underlying dermatitis/ eczema	Topical or systemic immunosuppressants	Sinus and fistula formation is associated with surgery (avoid surgery); treat with metronidazole and oral immunosuppressants

Additional reading

BASHH. UK National Guideline on the Management of Vulval Conditions. Clinical Effectiveness Group, British Association for Sexual Health and HIV. February 2014. https://www.bashh.org/documents/UK%20national%20 guideline%20for%20the%20management%20of%20vulval%20conditions%20 2014.pdf

Vulval skin disorders, management. Green-top Guideline No. 58. 2011. https:// www.rcog.org.uk/en/guidelines-research-services/guidelines/gtg58/

6. d

HPV TRIAGE

Women referred due to borderline/mild cytology or normal cytology/HPV positive, who then have a satisfactory and negative colposcopy can be recalled in 3 years. If the cytology sample is unreliable or inadequate for the HPV test, refer mild dyskaryosis for colposcopy and recall borderline for 6 months repeat cytology. At repeat cytology, an HPV test is performed if smear is negative, borderline or mild dyskaryosis. If HPV negative, then the patient can be returned to routine recall; refer to colposcopy if HPV positive. Refer moderate or worse cytology result for colposcopy.

HPV triage for low grade smears

Borderline or mild dyskaryosis	Borderline or mild dyskaryosis	Borderline or mild dyskaryosis	Borderline or mild dyskaryosis	Borderline or mild dyskaryosis	Borderline or mild dyskaryosis
HPV –ve →	HPV +ve →	HPV +ve →	HPV +ve →	HPV +ve →	HPV +ve →
Routine recall 3 or 5 yearly (depending on age <50 or >50 years	Refer to colposcopy → Colposcopy negative → Routine recall 3 or 5 yearly (depending on age <50 or >50 years	Refer to colposcopy → Colposcopy shows CIN1 → No treatment → Cytology at 12 months with or without colposcopy	Refer to colposcopy → Colposcopy shows CIN1 → Treatment undertaken → Normal cytology at 6 months and HPV –ve → 3-year recall cytology	Refer to colposcopy → Colposcopy shows CIN1 → Treatment undertaken → Normal cytology at 6 months and HPV+ve → Colposcopy and cytology follow-up as per national guidelines	Refer to colposcopy → Colposcopy shows CIN1 → Treatment undertaken → Abnormal cytology at 6 months → Colposcopy and cytology follow-up as per national guidelines

HPV triage and test of cure protocol

Borderline or mild dyskaryosis	Borderline or mild dyskaryosis	Borderline or mild dyskaryosis	Moderate or severe dyskaryosis	Moderate or severe dyskaryosis	Moderate or severe dyskaryosis
HPV +ve →	HPV +ve →	HPV +ve →	Refer to colposcopy →	Refer to colposcopy →	Refer to colposcopy →
Refer to colposcopy →	Refer to colposcopy →	Refer to colposcopy →	Treatment for CIN →	Treatment for CIN →	Treatment for CIN →
Colposcopy shows CIN2/3 →	Colposcopy shows CIN2/3 →	Colposcopy shows CIN2/3 →	Normal cytology at 6 months and HPV –ve →	Normal cytology at 6 months and HPV +ve →	Abnormal cytology at 6 months →
Treatment →	Treatment →	Treatment →	3-year recall cytology	Colposcopy and cytology follow-up as per national guidelines	Colposcopy and cytology follow-up as per national guidelines
Normal cytology at 6 months and HPV –ve →	Normal cytology at 6 months and HPV +ve →	Abnormal cytology at 6 months →			
3-year recall cytology	Colposcopy and cytology follow-up as per national guidelines	Colposcopy and cytology follow-up as per national guidelines			

Read NHSCSP algorithm. See additional references.

HPV test of cure following LLETZ

It will apply to all women attending their first post-treatment follow-up appointment or cytology test, irrespective of the grade of treated CIN, and all women in annual follow-up after treatment for CIN (wherever they are in the 10-year surveillance process). These women will then be managed in the same way, in accordance with the test of cure protocol.

All women entering the test of cure who have normal, borderline or mild cytology and are HR-HPV negative will be invited for their next cytology test in 3 years, regardless of their age. If at 3 years their cytology result is negative, women aged over 50 years should revert to their normal recall pattern (i.e. every 5 years). Women with moderate or worse cytology, whatever their age, will be referred to colposcopy.

If a woman fails to attend colposcopy following treatment and returns to the care of her GP before her first follow-up cytology, she should still be included in the test of cure protocol.

A woman will be referred to colposcopy if test of cure shows borderline changes or mild dyskaryosis or normal cytology and she is HR-HPV positive. If the colposcopy is satisfactory and negative she can be recalled in 3 years.

Women who reach the age of 65 years must be invited for screening until the protocol is complete, and otherwise comply with national guidance. Women aged over 60 who have borderline changes or mild dyskaryosis and test HR-HPV negative at triage can be ceased from the National Health Service Cervical Screening Programme (NHSCSP), as their next test due date would be after age 65. Women aged over 60 who have mild, borderline or normal cytology and are HR-HPV negative at test of cure will return for a further cytology test 3 years later, regardless of whether or not they will be aged over 65 when that test is due. Only if this further cytology test is normal can they be discharged from the programme. If a woman under the age of 25 years has received treatment for CIN she can be included in the HPV test of cure at her follow-up appointment, regardless of her age.

Additional reading

NHS Cervical Screening Programme. HPV triage and test of cure implementation guide. *NHSCSP good practice guide. No 3.* July 2011. http://www.csp.nhs.uk/files/F000198_F000196_NHSCSP%20Good%20Practice%20Guide%20no%203%20HPV%20implementation%20guidance.pdf

7. c

Women who carry *BRCA1* and *BRCA2* are at high risk of developing breast and ovarian cancers. The management of such women involves RRBSO and risk-reducing bilateral mastectomy or breast screening. With this prophylactic RRBSO, the risk of ovarian cancer is reduced by 80%–96% and breast cancer by 56% in women who carry *BRCA1* and 46% in women who carry *BRCA2*. (Also there is evidence that RRBSO improves survival and reduces mortality by 60%–76%.) However, women still have the risk of developing primary peritoneal carcinoma in 1%–6%, and this risk persists for up to 20 years after oophorectomy.

The risk of ovarian cancer increases significantly in her 40s for women who carry *BRCA1* and therefore RRBSO is recommended between 35 and 40 years of age. For women who carry *BRCA2*, the risk increases from mid-40s (from the age of 45 years) and therefore RRBSO can be delayed until 45 years of age.

There is no definite evidence that current screening methods for ovarian carcinoma improve survival in high-risk women. Currently, screening for ovarian carcinoma should not be an alternative RRBSO.

Additional reading

RCOG. Management of women with genetic predisposition to gynaecological cancers. *Scientific impact paper No 48*. February 2015.

8. c

FIGO classification of ovarian cancer (2014)	
Stage	Characteristics
I	Growth limited to ovaries
IA	Growth limited to one ovary. The ovarian capsule is intact without tumour on the external surface and no malignant cells present in washings or ascites
IB	Growth limited to both ovaries. The ovarian capsule is intact without tumour on the external surface and no malignant cells present in washings or ascites
IC	Either stage IA or IB but with tumour on the surface of one or both ovaries, or surgical spill, or capsule rupture before surgery or with ascites present containing cancerous cells, or with positive peritoneal washings
IC1	Surgical spill
IC2	Tumour on ovarian surface or capsule rupture before surgery
IC3	Positive peritoneal washings or ascites containing malignant cells
II	Growth involving one or both ovaries with spread to other pelvic organs (below the pelvic brim)
IIA	Metastasis to uterus or tubes
IIB	Metastasis to other pelvic intraperitoneal organs

Continued

FIGO classification of ovarian cancer (2014)	
Stage	Characteristics
III	Growth involving one or both ovaries with histologically or cytologically confirmed peritoneal implants outside the pelvis and/or positive retroperitoneal lymph nodes or omentum.
IIIA	Positive peritoneal spread confirmed microscopically or positive retroperitoneal lymph nodes
IIIA1	Positive retroperitoneal lymph nodes IIIA(i) – Metastasis less than 10 mm size IIIA(ii) – Metastasis more than 10 mm size
IIIA2	Microscopic peritoneal metastasis outside the pelvis ± positive retroperitoneal lymph nodes
IIIB	Macroscopic peritoneal metastasis <2 cm size outside the pelvis ± positive retroperitoneal lymph nodes ± involvement of liver and/or splenic capsule
IIIC	Macroscopic peritoneal metastasis >2 cm size outside the pelvis ± positive retroperitoneal lymph nodes ± involvement of liver and/or splenic capsule
IV	Distant metastasis excluding peritoneal metastasis
IVA	Analysis of pleural effusion showing malignant cells
IVB	Parenchymal liver and/or splenic metastasis and metastasis to extra-abdominal organs including inguinal lymph nodes and other lymph nodes outside the abdominal cavity

Five-year survival rates for ovarian cancer

FIGO Stage	Survival rate (%)
Stage 1	92
Stage 2	55
Stage 3	22
Stage 4	6
Overall survival for all stages	43

Additional reading

FIGO ovarian cancer staging. https://www.sgo.org/wp-content/uploads/2012/09/FIGO-Ovarian-Cancer-Staging_1.10.14.pdf

Cancer research UK. http://www.cancerresearchuk.org/cancer-info/cancerstats/types/ovary/

9. a

Endocervical gland involvement only is no longer stage II but will be stage I.

	FIGO classification of endometrial cancer
I	Tumour confined to uterus
IA	No or less than half myometrial invasion
IB	Invasion equal to or more than half of myometrium
II	Tumour involving the cervix stroma but does not extend outside the uterus
III	Local or regional spread of tumour outside the uterus
IIIA	Tumour involving the uterine serosa or adnexae
IIIB	Tumour involving vagina or parametrium
IIIC	Metastases to pelvic or para-aortic nodes
IIIC1	Metastases to pelvic nodes
IIIC2	Metastases to para-aortic nodes
IV	Tumour involves bladder or bowel mucosa or distant metastases
IVA	Tumour involves bladder or bowel mucosa
IVB	Distant metastasis involving intra-abdominal metastases and/or inguinal lymph nodes

Note: Endocervical gland involvement only is no longer stage II.

Positive cytology does not change the stage but is reported separately.

Endometrioid carcinoma can be grade 1, grade 2 or grade 3.

Five-year survival rates for endometrial cancer

FIGO Stage	Survival rate (%)
Stage 1	95
Stage 2	77
Stage 3	39
Stage 4	14
Overall survival for all stages	84.4

Additional reading

Endometrial cancer treatment. http://www.cancer.gov/cancertopics/pdq/treatment/endometrial/HealthProfessional/page3#_185_e

Cancer research UK. http://www.cancerresearchuk.org/cancer-info/cancerstats/types/uterus/survival/uterus-cancer-survival-statistics

FIGO committee on Gynaecologic Oncology. FIGO staging for carcinoma of the vulva, cervix, and corpus uteri. *International Journal of Gynaecology and Obstetrics.* 2014;125(2):97–8.

10. b

GRANULOSA CELL TUMOURS

This is a sex cord stromal tumour (malignant tumour) which occurs at the extremes of age (juvenile and adult types). They account for 70% of all stromal tumours. The average age at presentation is 52 years. Older women present with PMB while young girls present with menstrual problems or abnormal bleeding or precocious puberty. They typically produce oestrogen and cause endometrial hyperplasia and endometrial carcinoma (10% of cases). Most of these tumours are diagnosed at an early stage (stage I) and are generally unilateral. They spread similar to epithelial ovarian cancer. For stage I, the treatment is surgery and adjuvant therapy is not necessary. Stage II–IV cancers are treated with surgery and adjuvant chemotherapy. These tumours have a tendency to recur after a long time after clinical cure. Therefore, long-term follow-up is required in these patients. The prognosis for survival is generally good with 5-year survival rates around 80%. Advanced stage and recurrence are associated with high mortality.

Inhibin B levels (Alfa-subunit more specific) are measured at follow-up. The normal levels of inhibin in postmenopausal or oophorectomised women are less than or equal to 5 and 15 ng/L for inhibin A and inhibin B levels.

World Health Organisation (WHO) classification of non-epithelial ovarian cancer

Germ cell tumours
Dysgerminoma
Endodermal sinus tumour or yolk sac tumour
Embryonal carcinoma
Teratomas
Polyembryoma
Mixed type (two or more of the above types)
Gonadoblastoma (tumours composed of germ cells and sex cord stromal derivatives, e.g. Sertoli-Leydig)
Sex cord stromal tumours
Granulose cell tumour
Sertoli-stromal cell tumour
Gynandroblastoma
Unclassified
Metastatic tumours (Krukenberg)
Unclassified

Additional reading

Granulosa-theca cell tumour workup. http://emedicine.medscape.com/article/254489-workup

Sanusi FA, Carter P, Barton DPJ. Non-epithelial ovarian cancers. *The Obstetrician and Gynaecologist.* 2000;2(2).

Sourner P. The role of surgery in ovarian cancer. *RCOG Pace review No 97/10.*

TERATOMAS OF OVARY

Teratomas are germ cell tumours. They are classified as mature and immature teratomas. Mature teratomas are benign and arise from two or three germ cell layers. Rarely in 1%–2% of cases there is malignant transformation in mature teratomas (often this will be squamous cell carcinoma).

Immature teratomas are malignant tumours. They constitute 20% of germ cell tumours and 1% of ovarian cancer. They are almost always unilateral. They most commonly occur in the first two decades of life. They are derived from ectoderm, endoderm and mesoderm and contain both mature and immature elements (most often consisting of immature neural tissue). Specifically neurotubules and rosettes can be seen histologically. The tumour is graded histologically on the amount and degree of cellular immaturity particularly of neural tissue (graded as 1–3). The treatment includes surgery and chemotherapy. The tumour is not sensitive to radiotherapy. Grade 2 and grade 3 tumours are treated with adjuvant chemotherapy.

The prognostic factor for immature teratomas is different in children and adults. In children, the prognosis of immature teratomas depends on the presence or absence of yolk sac component.

Additional reading

Deodhar KK, Suryawanshi P, Shah M, Rekhi B, Chinoy RF. Immature teratoma of the ovary: A clinicopathological study of 28 cases. *Indian Journal of Pathology and Microbiology.* 2011 Oct–Dec;54(4):730–5.

Sanusi FA, Carter P, Barton DPJ. Non-epithelial ovarian cancers. *The Obstetrician and Gynaecologist.* April 2000;2(2).

Sourner P. The role of surgery in ovarian cancer. *RCOG Pace review No 97/10.*

12. d

KRUKENBERG TUMOUR (NAMED AFTER FRIEDRICH ERNST KRUKENBERG)

Metastatic tumour of the ovary accounts for only 1%–2% of ovarian cancer. The metastatic adenocarcinoma (named as Krukenberg tumour) usually arises from a primary malignancy of the gastrointestinal tract (76% originating from the stomach) or breast cancer (invasive lobular breast carcinoma). They can also arise in the appendix, small and large bowel, gallbladder, biliary tract and pancreas.

Krukenberg tumours are often bilateral (80%) and symmetrical in both ovaries. The histology shows mucin-secreting signet ring cells.

Additional reading

Sarris I et al. 2009. *Training in Obstetrics and Gynecology – The Essential Curriculum*. Oxford: Oxford University Press; 391–416.

13. d

FIGO classification of vulval carcinoma (2014)	
Stage	Characteristics
I	Tumour confined to vulva or perineum with negative nodes
IA	Tumour confined to the vulva or perineum, ≤2 cm in size with stromal invasion ≤1 mm, negative nodes
IB	Tumour confined to the vulva or perineum, >2 cm in size or with stromal invasion >1 mm, negative nodes
II	Tumour of any size with adjacent spread (one-third lower urethra, one-third lower vagina, anus), negative nodes
IIIA	Tumour of any size with positive inguino-femoral lymph nodes 1. One lymph node metastasis greater than or equal to 5 mm 2. One to two lymph node metastasis(es) of less than 5 mm
IIIB	1. Two or more lymph nodes metastases greater than or equal to 5 mm 2. Three or more lymph nodes metastases less than 5 mm
IIIC	Positive node(s) with extracapsular spread
IVA	1. Tumour invades other regional structures (two-thirds upper urethra, two-thirds upper vagina), bladder mucosa, rectal mucosa, or fixed to pelvic bone 2. Fixed or ulcerated inguino-femoral lymph nodes
IVB	Any distant metastasis including pelvic lymph nodes

Five-year survival rate for vulva cancer

FIGO Stage	Survival rate (%)
Stage 1	80
Stage 2	60
Stage 3	40
Stage 4	15

Note: Inguinal node status and spread to adjacent structures determine the survival in vulval cancer. In patients with nodal involvement, the 5-year overall survival (OS) is approximately 50%–60%. However, in patients with operable disease without nodal involvement, the OS rate is 90%.

Management of vulval carcinoma

Vulvar cancer accounts for about 4% of cancers in female reproductive organs and 0.6% of all cancers in women. Its incidence is increasing in young women because of its association with the HPV.

The treatment of vulval carcinoma must be individualised. The aim is cure of the disease with emphasis on a conservative surgical approach. When dealing with vulval cancer one has to remove the primary lesion as well as the groin lymph nodes.

Stage IA: Tumour confined to the vulva or perineum, ≤2 cm in size with stromal invasion ≤1 mm, negative nodes (the depth being measured from the epithelial-stromal junction of the most adjacent superficial dermal papilla to the deepest point of invasion). Such lesions should be managed with wide local excision. Groin dissection is not necessary for lesions of this type. Surgical margins should be at least 1 cm, and the deep margin should be the inferior fascia of the urogenital diaphragm.

Recurrence can occur in the groin and therefore should be addressed appropriately as per vulval stage. All patients with tumours >2 cm and all patients with tumours <2 cm with >1 mm depth of stromal invasion should have at least ipsilateral inguinofemoral lymphadenectomy. The incidence of contralateral node involvement in patients with T1 tumours (<2 m size) is <1%. Bilateral groin node dissection should be performed in women with midline tumours or those involving the clitoris.

Additional reading

FIGO Committee on Gynaecologic Oncology. FIGO staging for carcinoma of the vulva, cervix, and corpus uteri. *International Journal of Gynaecology and Obstetrics.* 2014;125(2):97–8.

Cancer research UK. http://www.cancerresearchuk.org/about-cancer/type/vulval-cancer/treatment/statistics-and-outlook-for-vulval-cancer

Homesley HD et al. Assessment of current International Federation of Gynecology and Obstetrics staging of vulvar carcinoma relative to prognostic factors for survival (a Gynecologic Oncology Group study). *American Journal of Obstetrics and Gynecology.* 164 (4):997–1003; discussion 1003–4, 1991.

14. b

All patients with moderate and severe dyskaryosis referred during pregnancy should have a colposcopy to rule out invasive disease. If feasible, they can have a repeat colposcopy during pregnancy.

Subsequently, these women should be followed up 3 months post-delivery as colposcopy can sometimes be difficult at this stage if the woman is still breastfeeding or her periods have not returned as the tissues are less well oestrogenised.

Additional reading

BSCCP webwise- NHSCSP-20 guidelines. https://www.gov.uk/government/uploads/system/uploads/attachment_data/file/436873/nhscsp20.pdf

15. c

RMI in her case is $30 \times 3 \times 3 = 270$. The risk of malignancy is significantly increased (>70%) if the RMI is >200. Therefore, she needs to be referred to the cancer centre.

Calculate the risk of malignancy index (RMI):RMI $= U \times M \times CA125$

$U = 0$ (for ultrasound score of 0); $U = 1$ (for ultrasound score of 1); $U = 3$ (for ultrasound score of 2–5). Ultrasound scans are scored one point for each of the following characteristics: multilocular cyst; evidence of solid areas; evidence of metastases; presence of ascites; and bilateral lesions.

$M = 3$ for all postmenopausal women dealt with by this guideline. CA125 is serum CA125 measurement in units/mL.

Additional reading

Management of ovarian cysts in postmenopausal women. *Green-top guideline No 34.*

16. e

Additional reading

Wheeless CR, Roenneburg ML. Radical Wertheim hysterectomy with bilateral pelvic lymph node dissection and with extension of the vagina. *Atlas of Pelvic Surgery (online edition).* http://www.atlasofpelvicsurgery.com/10MalignantDisease/15RadicalWertheimHysterectomyWithBilateralPelvicLymphNodeDissectionandWithExtensionoftheVagina/cha10sec15.html

17. b

FIGO STAGING OF CERVICAL CANCER

- IA1 Confined to the cervix, diagnosed only by microscopy with invasion of <3 mm in depth and lateral spread <7 mm
- IA2 Confined to the cervix, diagnosed with microscopy with invasion of >3 mm and <5 mm with lateral spread <7 mm
- IB1 Clinically visible lesion or greater than A2, <4 cm in greatest dimension
- IB2 Clinically visible lesion, >4 cm in greatest dimension
- IIA1 Involvement of the upper two-thirds of the vagina, without parametrial invasion, <4 cm in greatest dimension
- IIA2 >4 cm in greatest dimension
- IIB With parametrial involvement

Stage III Extends to the pelvic wall and/or involves the lower third of the vagina and/or causes hydronephrosis or non-functioning kidney.

- **IIIa** Lower third of the vagina
- **IIIb** pelvic wall and/or hydronephrosis or non-functioning kidney

Stage IV The carcinoma has extended beyond the true pelvis or has involved (biopsy proven) the mucosa of the bladder or rectum. A bullous edema, as such, does not permit a case to be allotted to stage IV.

- **IVa** Spread of the growth to adjacent organs
- **IVb** Spread to distant organs

Stage Ia1

- Women are diagnosed LLETZ or a cone biopsy.
- The incidence of lymph node involvement is <1%.
- If the excision margins are clear (invasive and pre-invasive) with 5 mm or more, no further treatment is necessary.
- If the excision margins are involved, further local excision should be performed.
- If simple hysterectomy is chosen in the presence of incomplete margins, a repeat loop or cone should be performed to exclude more extensive invasive disease that could necessitate a radical hysterectomy.

Additional reading

Cancer research UK. Treatment of cervical cancer. http://www.cancerresearchuk. org/about-cancer/cervical-cancer/treatment/treatment-decisions

GYNAECOLOGICAL PROBLEMS

Questions

1. A 40-year-old woman is referred to gynaecology clinic with large fibroids. Three are subserosal (5 × 6 cm, 6 × 5, 8 × 4 cm) and two are intramural (10 × 12 cm).

   Which one of the following would be a contraindication for uterine artery embolisation (UAE) in her case?
   a. Adenomyosis
   b. Menorrhagia
   c. Asymptomatic fibroids
   d. Presence of intrauterine copper device (IUCD)
   e. Woman who is a Jehovah's Witness

2. A 41-year-old woman presents with urinary frequency and pelvic pressure. An ultrasound scan reveals a large 20 cm intramural fibroid and four other small intramural fibroids. Urine dipstick test result was normal. She was reviewed in the gynaecology clinic and was offered myomectomy in view of her symptoms. The woman declines surgery but is willing to have UAE.

   Which statement is false regarding counselling of this patient?
   a. 1%–2% will have early ovarian failure
   b. May need further treatment in the form of hysterectomy in 2.9% of women
   c. 40%–70% reduction in the fibroid volume
   d. Risk of post-embolisation syndrome
   e. 98% of the patients will be symptom free following UAE

3. A 30-year-old woman presents to GP with increase in growth of hair on the chin, chest and back which she noticed for the last 3 months. She also gives history of deepening of voice and frontal hair loss. Vulval examination reveals clitoromegaly.

   Which one of the following tests differentiates androgen-producing adrenal tumour from ovarian tumour?
   a. Increased free serum testosterone levels
   b. Increased serum dehydroepiandrosterone (DHEA) levels
   c. Increased serum dehydroepiandrosterone sulphate (DHEAS) levels
   d. Decreased serum sex hormone binding globulin (SHBG) levels
   e. Increased serum 17-hydroxyprogesterone levels

4. A 30-year-old woman presents to GP with severe cyclical mastalgia. GP prescribes her Danazol 200 mg once daily for 3 months and arranges a follow-up after 3 months.

When counselling this woman one should explain the following except that it
a. Can cause osteoporosis with long-term use
b. Can cause irreversible changes in voice
c. Can cause virilisation of the female fetus if she gets pregnant
d. Can cause oily skin and acne
e. Should be avoided during pregnancy

5. One of the following is a recognised cause of gynaecomastia:
a. Charcot-Marie-Tooth syndrome
b. Down syndrome
c. Klinefelter syndrome
d. Lynch syndrome
e. Turner syndrome

6. Patient has an abnormal cervical smear and biopsy results are reported as high-grade cervical glandular intraepithelial neoplasia (CGIN).

This patient is at increased risk of
a. Endometrial carcinoma
b. Adenocarcinoma of cervix
c. Serous ovarian carcinoma
d. Endometrioid endometrial carcinoma
e. Cervical sarcoma

7. A 65-year-old, nulliparous woman presents to A&E with shortness of breath and cough. She is admitted under the acute medical team. Chest X-ray confirmed a right-sided pleural effusion. No malignant cells identified in the pleural aspirate. There was a large, firm abdominal mass palpated on examination of the abdomen with ascites.

What is the most likely explanation for this presentation?
a. Sheehan syndrome
b. Meigs syndrome
c. Atypical Meigs syndrome
d. Neuroendocrine carcinoma
e. Kikuchi disease

8. A 29-year-old, nulliparous woman presents with chronic pelvic pain. Her body mass index (BMI) is 45 and she gives history of midline laparotomy for ovarian cystectomy in the past. All her investigations including pelvic ultrasound and triple swabs are negative. You offer her a diagnostic laparoscopy with the intention to proceed if you find any pelvic pathology like endometriosis or adhesions.

The following risks are appropriate to discuss during consenting with this woman except
a. The overall risk of serious complications is 2/1000 women.
b. The risk of death is 100/100,000 because of complications.

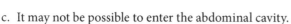

c. It may not be possible to enter the abdominal cavity.

d. It may not be possible to complete the procedure laparoscopically due to extensive adhesions.

e. Wound bruising may occur around the port sites.

9. A 70-year-old woman with history of vaginal prolapse is referred to the gynaecology clinic by GP. Pelvic examination reveals procidentia. General examination reveals clear fluid-filled dome-shaped firm blisters on the arm, legs and bilateral groin. Her previous clinic letter reveals that she has been on long-term steroids for this condition. You see scarring of the previous blisters on the arm and legs. Previous biopsy and immunofluorescence studies show antibody deposits at dermo-epidermal junction.

What is the most likely diagnosis of the skin condition in her case?
a. Pemphigus vulgaris
b. Bullous pemphigoid
c. Psoriasis
d. Erythema multiforme
e. Dermatitis herpetiformis

10. Intralipid is made up of all of the following except
a. Soybean oil
b. Egg yolk phospholipids
c. Glycerin
d. Sodium
e. Water

11. The following risks have been reported regarding administration of Intralipid other than
a. Hypercoagulation
b. Severe sepsis
c. Disseminated intravascular coagulation (DIC)
d. Allergic reaction
e. Fetal teratogenicity

12. Intralipid use has been reported to be of benefit in one of the following conditions:
a. Assisted conception
b. Recurrent miscarriage
c. Disseminated intravascular coagulation
d. Local anaesthetic toxicity
e. Anaphylaxis to intravenous iron

13. A 45-year-old woman is referred to gynaecology clinic with history of menorrhagia, dysmenorrhoea and past history of premenstrual syndrome. Her haemoglobin is 11 gm% and pelvic ultrasound scan is normal. All the options of management are discussed with her in the clinic by specialist registrar. She wishes to have endometrial ablation for treatment.

All the statements regarding her counselling this woman are true except
a. Subsequent pregnancy should be avoided.
b. Further contraception will be necessary.

c. Dysmenorrhoea will be relieved.

d. Premenstrual syndrome will not be relieved.

e. Approximately 20% will have no benefit with endometrial ablation.

14. A 42-year-old woman with abnormal vaginal bleeding has an endometrial Pipelle biopsy. The histology shows endometrial hyperplasia.

To treat her appropriately the following need to be determined except for

a. The type of hyperplasia

b. Malignant potential

c. Fertility wishes

d. Sources of any exogenous (e.g. tamoxifen) and endogenous (ovarian tumour) oestrogen

e. Ethnic origin

15. A 44-year-old woman is referred to a menopausal clinic with severe vasomotor symptoms and low mood. She has a history of oestrogen-receptor-positive and progesterone-receptor-negative breast cancer which was treated with wide local excision and radiotherapy. She is currently on tamoxifen.

What would you prescribe to treat her menopausal symptoms?

a. Selective serotonin reuptake inhibitors (SSRIs)

b. Conjugated equine oestrogens

c. Oestrogen and PG

d. Topical vaginal oestrogen

e. Clonidine

16. A 38-year-old woman is referred to gynaecology clinic by GP. She gives history of amenorrhoea for the past 6 months. She has two children delivered by caesarean section and regular periods prior to this. Her urine pregnancy test is negative. Her mother had premature menopause at the age of 30.

The diagnosis in her case is based on

a. Single elevated follicle-stimulating hormone (FSH) levels on blood test

b. Elevated anti-müllerian hormone levels and inhibin A levels on blood test

c. Elevated inhibin A levels on blood test

d. Elevated FSH levels on two blood samples taken 4–6 weeks apart

e. Single elevated FSH levels and anti-müllerian hormone levels on blood test

17. A 37-year-old woman, para 1 is referred to gynaecology clinic as a 2 weeks' wait in view of abdominal swelling and pelvic pressure. An ultrasound scan attached with GP referral shows a large uterus (uterine size of 20×10 cm) with multiple fibroids. She wishes to have uterine artery embolisation.

Which of the following is not an absolute contraindication for uterine artery embolisation?

a. Asymptomatic fibroids in women <40 years of age

b. Infection of the genital tract 3 weeks ago

c. Pedunculated fibroid

d. Sixteen weeks' pregnancy

e. Where a patient would refuse a hysterectomy under any circumstances due to social or cultural reasons even after appropriate counselling

Answers

1. c

UTERINE ARTERY EMBOLISATION (UAE)

Indications

UAE is indicated in women with symptomatic fibroids (causing heavy periods, dysmenorrhoea, pain, dyspareunia and pressure symptoms on bowel or bladder). It can be used in women with adenomyosis although it is reported to be less efficacious (women should be counselled appropriately). If surgery is contraindicated (e.g. Jehovah's Witness or women who had previous unsuccessful surgery for fibroids), UAE can be considered.

Absolute contraindications

- Asymptomatic fibroids
- Recent or current infection of the genital tract
- Pregnancy
- If the diagnosis is uncertain due to clinical factors or inadequate imaging
- When patient declines hysterectomy due to social or cultural reasons even after appropriate counselling (small proportion of the patients need hysterectomy following UAE)

Relative contraindications

- Narrow stalk pedunculated submucous fibroid (can get detached and block the cervical canal)
- Large intracavitary submucous fibroid (may result in sloughing of the fibroid and cause cervical obstruction and occasional sepsis)
- Pedunculated subserosal fibroids (may detach the pedicle and may need laparoscopic removal of these fibroids)
- If woman wants to preserve fertility and has symptomatic fibroids (ovarian failure can occur in 1%–2% although more common in women over 45 years and those who are nearing menopause)

Additional reading

Royal College of Radiologists (RCR) and Royal College of Obstetricians and Gynaecologists (RCOG). *Clinical Recommendations on the Use of Uterine Artery Embolisation (UAE) in the Management of Fibroids*, 3rd ed. 2013. https://www.rcog.org.uk/globalassets/documents/guidelines/23-12-2013_rcog_rcr_uae.pdf

2. e

UTERINE ARTERY EMBOLISATION (UAE)

At 1 year, 80%–90% of the patients will be asymptomatic or have significantly improved symptoms.

Counselling of the patient should include discussion of the procedure as well as risks. The risks of the procedure include

- Puncture site bruising
- Self-limiting vaginal discharge (20%–30% of patients)
- Passage of fibroid material (6% of patients will require additional procedure to remove them)
- Amenorrhoea occurs in 1.5%–7% of patients but is dependent on age
- Ovarian dysfunction
- Emergency hysterectomy in 1% (may occur months after UAE)
- Recurrence of symptoms and need for further treatment
- (By 5 years, the risk is 25% in women less than 40 years of age and 10% between 40 and 50 years of age).
- Effects of UAE on fertility and pregnancy are uncertain

Complications of UAE

Immediate	Early (within 30 days)	Late (after 30 days)
Arterial thrombosis	Post-embolisation syndrome (pain, nausea, fever and malaise)	Vaginal discharge (16% at 12 months). It is common and self-limiting.
Groin haematoma	Infection and readmission in 3%–5% of patients	Foul-smelling discharge is due to infection and should be treated. If not responding to treatment, magnetic resonance imaging should be performed to exclude pelvic abscess, fibroid impaction and retained fragments of tissue.
Dissection and pseudoaneurysm	Urinary tract infection – very rare	Persistent vaginal discharge – rule out fibroid expulsion.
Allergic reaction to contrast media	Deep venous thrombosis – very rare	Fibroid expulsion and impaction occurs in 10% and is more common with submucous fibroids.
Uterine artery spasm and incomplete embolisation		Non-target embolisation of ovarian artery may lead to amenorrhoea. Incidence at 12 months 1.5%–7% (<1% in women below 40 years of age and 8% in women over 45 years age).
Non-target embolisation (particles reaching other vascular beds)		Endometritis occurs in 0.5% of cases and requires antibiotic administration and intravenous (IV) fluids.
		Emergency hysterectomy may be required for severe sepsis following UAE.

Additional reading

Royal College of Radiologists (RCR) and Royal College of Obstetricians and
Gynaecologists (RCOG). *Clinical Recommendations on the Use of Uterine
Artery Embolisation (UAE) in the Management of Fibroids.* 3rd ed. 2013.
https://www.rcog.org.uk/globalassets/documents/guidelines/23-12-2013_
rcog_rcr_uae.pdf

3. c

Androgen-secreting tumours are generally associated with rapidly progressive
symptoms of hyperandrogenism, which can result in virilisation. A normal
DHEAS with increased plasma concentration of testosterone of more than
8.7 nmol/L (two to three times the normal value) is highly suggestive of an ovarian
androgen-secreting tumour. Both testosterone and DHEAS will be increased in
adrenal tumours (DHEAS exclusively produced in the adrenal gland). Although
a dexamethasone test is highly sensitive to it, that test has limited specificity
in differential diagnosis of hyperandrogenism. Ovarian and adrenal venous
catheterisation and sampling should be reserved for patients in whom imaging
studies cannot exclude a small ovarian tumour. The prognosis for ovarian
androgen-secreting tumour is generally good.

Hirsutism refers to male-pattern body hair (e.g. beard or hair on the
chest). Virilisation is associated development of male secondary sexual
characteristics.

Causes of hirsutism

Ovary	Adrenal gland	External causes
Polycystic ovary syndrome (PCOS) 95%	Congenital adrenal hyperplasia (CAP) <1%	Iatrogenic hirsutism <1%
Androgen-secreting tumour <1%	Cushing syndrome <1%	Drugs with androgenic effect (anabolic steroids, danazol,
Luteoma of pregnancy <1%	Androgen-secreting tumour <1%	testosterone) <1%

Pathophysiology of hirsutism

Increased exposure to androgen		Increased end-organ sensitivity	

Exogenous androgens	Androgens
	Progestogens with
	  androgenic potential
	Danazol
	Testosterone
		5-alpha reductase
		  activity in the skin
			Insulin growth factor in
			patients with insulin
			resistance and
			hyperinsulinaemia

Increased
production
	Tumours
	Enzyme defects (CAP)
	Cushing syndrome
	  Hyperinsulinaemia
	  Increased luteinizing
	  hormone (LH) levels
	Stimulate theca cells		

Alterations in binding globulins (SHBG)	Hyperinsulinaemia Liver disease Androgens Hyperprolactinemia Hypothyroidism		

Investigations

- Testosterone levels (produced both in ovary and testis)
- DHEAS (exclusively produced in the adrenal gland)
- Oral glucose tolerance test (OGTT) – insulin resistance (seen in PCOS)
- 17-Hydroxyprogesterone (rule out congenital adrenal hyperplasia)
- 24-Hour urinary cortisol levels, early morning serum cortisol before 9 a.m. and dexamethasone suppression test (rule out Cushing syndrome)
- Transvaginal scan (TVS) to rule out any ovarian pathology
- Abdominal scan to rule any adrenal mass

Additional reading

Collins S et al. *Oxford Handbook of Obstetrics and Gynaecology.* 3rd ed. Oxford: Oxford University Press, 2013.
Available at: http://eknygos.lsmuni.lt/springer/516/75-84.pdf

DANAZOL

It is a derivative of the synthetic steroid ethisterone that inhibits ovarian responsiveness and steroidogenesis. (It suppresses the mid-cycle LH surge, reduces LH pulsatility.) It is fat soluble and isoxazole of testosterone and exhibits hyperandrogenic effects that cause atrophy of the endometrium. It does not have either oestrogenic or progestogenic effects. It displaces testosterone from SHBG and reduces the hepatic synthesis of SHBG, hence increases the free serum testosterone levels resulting in androgenic side effects.

It has been used to treat severe cystic mastalgia, premenstrual syndrome (PMS) and menorrhagia. Sustained improvement is seen for several months after treatment in cystic mastalgia. It is superior to placebo in the treatment of PMS. The dose used is 100–400 mg once daily for 2–4 months. Evidence suggests that the use of danazol in patients with infertility and mild endometriosis does not benefit in increasing the pregnancy rate. One should use reliable contraception while using danazol as it can cause virilization of the female fetus if the woman gets pregnant.

The side effects include oily skin, acne, hirsutism (increase in facial hair), deepening of the voice (can be irreversible) and adverse blood lipid profile. It can also cause hot flushes, elevated liver enzymes and mood changes. It does not cause osteoporosis unlike gonadotropin-releasing hormone (GNRH) analogues. Some patients may complain of fluid retention and weight gain. In view of its side effects, it is not recommended to be used for more than 6 months.

Additional reading

Collins S et al. *Oxford Handbook of Obstetrics and Gynaecology.* 3rd ed. Oxford: Oxford University Press, 2013.

5. c

Gynaecomastia is defined as benign proliferation of the male glandular breast tissue. It is usually bilateral. It is associated with a relative excess of oestrogen compared with testosterone (increased oestrogen activity, decreased testosterone activity, drug therapies or decreased catabolism of oestrogen in the body).

The causes of gynaecomastia include

- Idiopathic (58%)
- Hypogonadism (25%)
- Chronic liver disease (4%)
- Hyperprolactinemia (9%)
- Drug induced (4%)
- Hyperthyroidism

Spironolactone (anti-androgen) used to treat hypertension and hyperandrogenic conditions can cause gynaecomastia (other drugs include flutamide and finasteride).One of the characteristic features of Klinefelter syndrome (47 XXY) is gynaecomastia. Oestrogen is metabolised in the liver which can be affected in liver cirrhosis resulting in increased serum oestrogen levels.

Prognosis is usually good as this is a self-limiting condition. Oestrogen receptor modifiers have been used in its treatment. Surgery is the standard treatment for gynaecomastia.

Additional reading

Ersöz H, Onde ME, Terekeci H, Kurtoglu S, Tor H. Causes of gynaecomastia in young adult males and factors associated with idiopathic gynaecomastia. *International Journal of Andrology.* 2002;25(5):312–6.

Ruth E. Johnson M, Murad H. Gynecomastia: Pathophysiology, evaluation, and management. *Mayo Clinic Proceedings.* 2009;84(11):1010–15. Available at: http://www.ncbi.nlm.nih.gov/pmc/articles/PMC2770912/

6. b

CERVICAL GLANDULAR INTRAEPITHELIAL NEOPLASIA (CGIN)

CGIN is a premalignant glandular cervical lesion and affects the columnar cells in the endocervical canal. It coexists with cervical intraepithelial lesions (squamous) in 50% of cases and therefore pure disease is uncommon. Glandular abnormalities of the cervix are relatively rare and account for only 0.05% (1 in 2,000) of cytological abnormalities. CGIN has an uncertain natural history unlike squamous lesions. The screening programme mainly aims at detecting squamous and not glandular lesions.

The National Health Service Cervical Screening Programme (NHSCSP) publication recommends urgent colposcopy referral after one test is reported as possible glandular neoplasia (100%) as the natural history of this condition is unclear. All women should be seen in the colposcopy clinic within 2 weeks of receipt of referral as there is increased risk of an underlying (cervical) malignancy (40%). It can be associated with underlying adenocarcinoma in the cervix, endometrium and very rarely in the ovary.

CGIN is multifocal in 15% of cases (skip lesions), and this has implications for diagnosis (unsatisfactory colposcopy) and treatment. Even with presumed adequate treatment with clear margins the risk of recurrence is high (15% with cervical glandular intraepithelial neoplasia [CGIN] and 5% with cervical intraepithelial neoplasia [CIN]). Almost 50% of CGIN are associated with high-grade CIN. The presence of squamous lesions should be taken into account in managing these cases. Ninety-five per cent (95%) of the CGIN extends within 25 mm of the anatomical external os. Despite originating from the columnar cells, 85% of the CGIN are found in the transformation zone (TZ) and deep clefts up to 5 mm from the margin of the canal can be involved.

One needs to counsel the women regarding the multifocal nature of this condition, high recurrence rate (15% by 4 years) and need for further treatment in one-fifth of the cases. Also, one needs to explain the high false-positive rate of glandular abnormality in cervical cytology and consequent negative biopsy on histology. If the margins of the first cone biopsy are not clear, it is reasonable to offer a repeat cone biopsy in order to exclude invasion and obtain negative margins. A hysterectomy (preferably vaginally) should be offered if she has completed her family or does not wish to conceive in the future. Close surveillance for 10 years of conservatively treated women should consist of cytology (with endocervical brush) and may be best managed in colposcopy clinic.

Additional reading

NHS Cervical Screening Programme. Colposcopy and Programme Management. *Guidelines for the NHS Cervical Screening Programme.* 2nd ed. Publication No 20. NHSCSP, 2010. http://www.bsccp.org.uk/docs/public/pdf/nhscsp20.pdf

Sarris I et al. *Training in Obstetrics and Gynecology – The Essential Curriculum.* Oxford: Oxford University Press, 2009, 391–416.

7. b

Meigs syndrome: The three typical features of Meigs syndrome include a benign tumour, ascites and right-sided pleural effusion. It is uncommon before the age of 40 and is usually associated with fibroma. It may also be associated with thecoma or fibro-thecoma of the ovary. As it is a benign condition, the prognosis is good. The symptoms (pressure symptoms) and ascites and effusion usually resolve once the tumour is removed.

Pseudo-Meigs syndrome: It is characterised by ascites, pleural effusion and benign ovarian tumours (other than fibromas). These include mature teratomas, struma ovarii or ovarian leiomyomas.

Atypical Meigs syndrome: It is associated with benign pelvic mass with a right-sided pleural effusion but no ascites.

Additional reading

Sarris I et al. *Training in Obstetrics and Gynecology – The Essential Curriculum.* Oxford: Oxford University Press, 2009, 391–416.

8. b

LAPAROSCOPIC SURGERY: CONSENTING AND RISKS OF SURGERY

Risks of laparoscopic surgery

- The overall risk of serious complications is 2/1,000 women (include damage to the bowel, bladder, ureter and major blood vessels which may need laparotomy to repair the damage). However, 15% of the bowel injuries are not recognised at the time of surgery and may present later.
- The risk of death is 8/100,000 because of complications and is not routinely discussed by doctors during consent.
- It may not be possible to enter the abdominal cavity (especially in women with a high BMI).
- There is risk of hernia at the port sites. Therefore, a lateral port more than 7 mm in size and central ports >10 mm should be closed with a J-shaped needle.
- The risk of frequent complications includes shoulder tip pain (due to leftover gas in the abdomen irritating the diaphragm), wound bruising, gaping and infection.
- The additional procedures one should discuss include laparotomy, rectification of serious complications (e.g. repair of damage to bowel, bladder, ureter and vessels) and blood transfusion.

Methods to minimise risks

- Medically, she should have anti-embolism (T.E.D.) stockings and Flowtron system if the duration of surgery is going to be more than 1 hour.
- One can possibly postpone the surgery if BMI is high (optimise BMI before surgery).
- Use Palmer's entry instead of umbilical entry as there is risk of midline adhesions and damage to the bowel.
- The length of the trocars can be 100 mm instead of 75 mm so the length is appropriate for the depth of the abdominal wall.
- The woman should be clearly warned about failure to enter the abdomen due to high BMI and therefore failure to complete the procedure laparoscopically.
- Laparotomy is associated with increased morbidity in women with high BMI.
- Postoperatively, good pain relief is important as it will promote early mobilisation and discharge from the hospital.

Additional reading

Royal College of Obstetricians and Gynaecologists (RCOG). *Green-Top Guideline No. 2. Diagnostic Laparoscopy.* London: RCOG Press, 2008.

9. b

Difference between bullous pemphigoid and pemphigus vulgaris

Bullous pemphigoid	Pemphigus vulgaris
Occurs in older women	Occurs in young
Rare on vulva	Rare on vulva
Subepidermal blistering	Intraepidermal blistering
Lesions heal with scarring	Lesions heal without scarring
In pemphigoid, this is due to anti-hemidesmosome antibodies and the detachment occurs between the epidermis and dermis (subepidermal bullae)	Transudate fluid accumulates in between the keratinocytes and basement membrane (supra-basal split) forming blister (Nikolsky sign)
Microscopy: shows subepidermal blister with inflammatory infiltrate (typically polymorphous with an eosinophilic predominance (mast cells and basophils may be prominent during early course of disease)	Microscopy: shows detachment of keratinocytes from each other due to loss of desmosome integrity causing acantholysis and intradermal bulla formation
Immunofluorescence studies on biopsies of lesions show antibody deposits at dermo-epidermal junction	Immunofluorescence studies on biopsies of lesions show antibody deposits at intercellular spaces of the epidermis
Direct immunofluorescent staining in bullous pemphigoid usually demonstrates immunoglobulin G (IgG) in 90% and C3 complement (in 100%) deposition in a linear band at the dermo-epidermal junction	Direct immunofluorescent staining shows acantholytic cells. These cells are basically rounded, nucleated keratinocytes formed due to antibody-mediated damage to cell adhesion protein desmoglein.
Serum studies: show the presence of circulating serum IgG auto-antibodies that target the skin basement membrane component (70% patients with bullous pemphigoid will have auto-antibodies that bind to split skin)	

Systemic immunosuppressive therapy and oral corticosteroids are usually required to prevent scarring.

Additional reading

Nunns D, Scott IV. Ulcers and erosions of the vulva. Personal assessment in continuing education. *Reviews, Questions and Answers*. RCOG Press, Feb 2003.
http://www.niams.nih.gov/Health_Info/Pemphigus/#7

10. e

INTRALIPID

Intralipid (20%) is a sterile, non-pyrogenic fat emulsion prepared for intravenous administration as a source of calories and essential fatty acids. It is made up of 20% soybean oil, 1.2% egg yolk phospholipids, 2.25% glycerine and water for injection.

Additional reading

Royal College of Obstetricians and Gynaecologists (RCOG). *Green-top Guideline No. 56. Maternal Collapse in Pregnancy and Peurperium.* London: RCOG Press, 2011.

11. d

RISK REGARDING INTRALIPID

A recent letter from the president of Royal College of Obstetricians and Gynaecologists (RCOG) reports cases of severe sepsis which have been attributed to poor practice in the administration leading to contamination of the product.

Cases of DIC have been reported in the literature. So far neither carcinogenic nor mutagenic effect has been assessed. It is not known whether Intralipid can cause harm to fetus when administered to pregnant women or if it can affect fertility (no animal studies reported as per U.S. Food and Drug Administration [FDA]).

Additional reading

Royal College of Obstetricians and Gynaecologists (RCOG). *Green-top Guideline No. 56. Maternal Collapse in Pregnancy and Peurperium.* London: RCOG Press, 2011.

12. d

USES OF INTRALIPID

In obstetrics, it is mainly used for the treatment for local anaesthetic toxicity (lignocaine). It can also be used to treat toxicity due to other lipid-soluble drugs. Intralipid preparations have been used for parenteral nutrition to deliver essential fatty acids. There is no evidence to suggest its use in assisted reproduction or recurrent miscarriage.

Additional reading

Royal College of Obstetricians and Gynaecologists (RCOG). *Green-top Guideline No. 56. Maternal Collapse in Pregnancy and Peurperium.* London: RCOG Press, 2011.

13. c

ENDOMETRIAL ABLATION

Endometrial ablation techniques destroy the endometrium. It can be performed by resectoscopic techniques or non-resectoscopic techniques.

Pre-requisites prior to performing endometrial ablation

- Urine pregnancy test
- Endometrial biopsy to rule out endometrial cancer
- Removal of intrauterine coil if there is one
- If possible thin the endometrium by progestogens or curettage of the uterus as this increases the success rate of the ablation if the endometrium is thin (with resectoscopic endometrial ablation, the rate of amenorrhoea with prior endometrial thinning were 39% with GnRH (gonadotrophin releasing hormones), 34% with danazol, 26% with medroxyprogesterone acetate and 18% with dilatation and curettage)

Types of ablation procedures for the endometrium

- Electrosurgery
- Cryotherapy where extreme cold is used to destroy the endometrium
- Uterine balloon inflated with hot fluid
- Microwave ablation
- Radiofrequency ablation

Indications for endometrial ablations

- Heavy menstrual bleeding due to benign condition
- Failure of medical therapy
- Patient who decline major surgery or high risk for surgery or not fit for major surgery

Contraindications for endometrial ablation

- Desiring fertility preservation
- Suspected hyperplasia or cancer of uterus
- Cervical cancer
- Current pelvic infection
- Procedure specific contraindications

Precautions and advise to patients

Endometrial ablation does not provide contraception for women. Therefore they need to be advised regarding using contraception and more so reliable contraception in view that if a woman gets pregnant these pregnancies may be at higher risk for the mother and the baby (increased risk of miscarriage and also ectopic pregnancies).

What to expect after the procedure?

- Abdominal cramps for few days
- Vaginal watery discharge

The most common endometrial ablation procedure used in UK is Novasure procedure. It is a quick procedure which takes less than five minutes and does not require general anaesthesia. Following the procedure 40% will have complete amenorrhoea and 90% will have light, normal or no periods.

Serious complications of endometrial ablation

- Uterine peroration: 0.3% for non-resectoscopic and 1.3% for resectoscopic endometrial ablations.
- Peri-operative haemorrhage: 1.2% for non-resectoscopic and 3% for resectoscopic endometrial ablation.
- Haematometra: 0.9% for non-resectoscopic and 2.4% for resectoscopic endometrial ablation.
- Post ablation tubal sterilization syndrome: 10% risk (cyclical or intermittent pelvic pain in women who have had prior tubal sterilization).
- Pelvic infection and fever: 1%
- Intra-uterine adhesions.
- Long term recurrent bleeding: may be due to endometrial regeneration or other pathology such as adenomyosis or fibroids. However if the ablation is more than a year and the bleeding persists, an endometrial biopsy is warranted

to exclude endometrial hyperplasia or endometrial cancer. If adequate sample cannot be obtained due to intrauterine adhesions which are often the case, a hysterectomy should be offered to these women.

Additional reading

Collins S et al. *Oxford Handbook of Obstetrics and Gynaecology.* 3rd ed. Oxford: Oxford University Press, 2013.

National Institute for Health and Care Excellence (NICE). Heavy menstrual bleeding: Assessment and management. *NICE guidelines (CG44):* January 2007.

Shawki O, Peters A, Abraham-Hebert S. Hysteroscopic endometrial destruction, optimum method for preoperative endometrial preparation: A prospective, randomized, multicenter evaluation. *JSLS.* 2002;6:23–7.

SOGC Clinical Practice Guideline. Endometrial ablation in the management of abnormal uterine bleeding. No. 322. April 2015.

https://sogc.org/wp-content/uploads/2015/04/GUI322CPG1504E2.pdf

https://www.webmd.com/women/endometriosis/what-is-endometrial-ablation#1

14. e

ENDOMETRIAL HYPERPLASIA

Endometrial hyperplasia (EH) is usually detected following investigation for abnormal uterine bleeding. This can occur in pre- and postmenopausal women.

Risk factors

- Unopposed oestrogen therapy
- Obesity (BMI >35)
- Nulliparity
- Diabetes
- Tamoxifen
- PCOS (anovulation)
- Oestrogen-secreting tumours (e.g. ovarian granulosa cell tumour)

Revised 2014 World Health Organization classification risk of malignant potential

- Hyperplasia without atypia
- Atypical hyperplasia: risk of (the complexity of architecture is no longer part of the classification)

One must take into account the following factors to decide about appropriate management

- Type of hyperplasia
- Fertility wishes
- Medical co-morbidities
- Risk of cancer progression

Initial management of women with EH without atypia

- EH progressing to cancer is less than 5% over 20 years
- Majority spontaneously regress
- Identify and modify risk – obesity/hormone replacement therapy (HRT)
- 10% obese women harbour asymptomatic EH
- Treatment with PGs – higher rate of disease regression (89%–96%) compared with observation alone (74%–81%)
- PG indicated if does not regress with observation alone or symptomatic women with abnormal bleeding

First-line medical treatment of hyperplasia without atypia

- Both continuous oral and local intrauterine (levonorgestrel-releasing intrauterine system [LNG-IUS]) PGs are effective in achieving regression of endometrial hyperplasia without atypia.
- Relapse is more common with oral PGs.
- The LNG-IUS should be the first-line medical treatment because compared with oral PGs it has a higher disease regression rate with a more favourable bleeding profile, and it is associated with fewer adverse effects.
- IUS – minimum 6/12 for histological regression; retain for 5 years.
- Endometrial surveillance at 6-monthly intervals – need at least two consecutive negative biopsies before discharge.
- Continuous PGs should be used (medroxyprogesterone 10–20 mg/day or norethisterone 10–15 mg/day) for women who decline the LNG-IUS.
- Cyclical PGs should not be used because they are less effective in inducing regression of endometrial hyperplasia without atypia compared with continuous oral PGs or the LNG-IUS.

Duration of treatment and follow-up of hyperplasia without atypia

- Treatment with oral PGs or the LNG-IUS should be for a minimum of 6 months in order to induce histological regression of endometrial hyperplasia without atypia. If adverse effects are tolerable and fertility is not desired, women should be encouraged to retain the LNG-IUS for up to 5 years as this reduces the risk of relapse, especially if it alleviates abnormal uterine bleeding symptoms.
- Endometrial surveillance incorporating outpatient endometrial biopsy is recommended after a diagnosis of hyperplasia without atypia. Endometrial

surveillance should be arranged at a minimum of 6-monthly intervals, although review schedules should be individualised and responsive to changes in a woman's clinical condition.

- At least two consecutive 6-monthly negative biopsies should be obtained prior to discharge. Women should be advised to seek a further referral if abnormal vaginal bleeding recurs after completion of treatment because this may indicate disease relapse.
- In women at higher risk of relapse, such as women with a BMI of 35 or greater or those treated with oral PGs, 6-monthly endometrial biopsies are recommended. Once two consecutive negative endometrial biopsies have been obtained then long-term follow-up should be considered with annual endometrial biopsies.
- If the hyperplasia persists for 12 months despite treatment or if there is progression during follow-up or there is persistence of abnormal vaginal bleeding, or there is relapse of endometrial hyperplasia following PG treatment or the women declines surveillance or does not comply with treatment, then hysterectomy should be considered as there is significant risk of progression to endometrial cancer.

Endometrial hyperplasia with atypia

- 8% risk of progression to cancer in 4 years
- 12% risk of progression to cancer after 9 years
- 27.5% risk of progression to cancer after 19 years
- Associated with carcinoma in situ in up to 43% of women undergoing hysterectomy
- Avoid morcellation
- Do not do supravesical hysterectomy
- No need for lymph node dissection - low risk for lymph node involvement as even if cancer is seen in the final histology at hysterectomy, these are low grade and early stage endometriod endometrial carcinoma.

Treatment of women with endometrial hyperplasia with atypia

- The risk of cancer progression or persistence is high with atypical hyperplasia (30%–50%).
- The risk of concurrent endometrial cancer with complex atypical hyperplasia is up to 40%. Therefore, a further hysteroscopy and thorough endometrial sampling should be considered despite diagnosis of hyperplasia on endometrial Pipelle biopsy.
- Women with atypical hyperplasia should undergo a total hysterectomy because of the risk of underlying malignancy or progression to cancer.
- Postmenopausal women with atypical hyperplasia should be offered bilateral salpingo-oophorectomy together with the total hysterectomy.
- For premenopausal women, the decision to remove the ovaries should be individualised; however, bilateral salpingectomy should be considered as this may reduce the risk of a future ovarian malignancy.

- A laparoscopic approach to total hysterectomy is preferable to an abdominal approach as it is associated with a shorter hospital stay, less postoperative pain and quicker recovery.
- There is no benefit from intraoperative frozen section analysis of the endometrium or routine lymphadenectomy.
- Postmenopausal women with atypical hyperplasia should be offered bilateral salpingo-oophorectomy together with the total hysterectomy.
- For premenopausal women, the decision to remove the ovaries should be individualised; however, bilateral salpingectomy should be considered as this may reduce the risk of a future ovarian malignancy.
- Endometrial ablation is not recommended because complete and persistent endometrial destruction cannot be ensured and intrauterine adhesion formation may preclude endometrial histological surveillance.
- Women wishing to retain the infertility should be counselled about the risks of underlying malignancy and subsequent progression to endometrial cancer.
- Pretreatment investigations should aim to rule out invasive endometrial cancer or co-existing ovarian cancer.
- Histology, imaging and tumour marker results should be reviewed in a multidisciplinary meeting and a plan for management and ongoing endometrial surveillance formulated.
- In women who wish to preserve fertility, first-line treatment with the LNG-IUS should be recommended, with oral PGs as a second-best alternative.
- With atypia it is necessary to treat women with LNG-IUS and high-dose oral PGs together in women who decline to have hysterectomy and perform hysteroscopy and endometrial biopsy at 6 months follow-up to check persistence or regression with this treatment.
- Once fertility is no longer required, hysterectomy should be offered in view of the high risk of disease relapse.

How should women with atypical hyperplasia not undergoing hysterectomy be followed up?

Routine endometrial surveillance should include endometrial biopsy. Review schedules should be individualised and be responsive to changes in a woman's clinical condition. Review intervals should be every 3 months until two consecutive negative biopsies are obtained. In asymptomatic women with a uterus and evidence of histological disease regression, based upon a minimum of two consecutive negative endometrial biopsies, long-term follow-up with endometrial biopsy every 6–12 months is recommended until a hysterectomy is performed.

How should endometrial hyperplasia be managed in women wishing to conceive?

- Disease regression on at least one sample
- Referral to fertility specialist

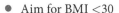
- Aim for BMI <30
- Assisted reproduction – live birth rate higher and can prevent relapse

Assisted reproduction may be considered as the live birth rate is higher and it may prevent relapse compared with women who attempt natural conception. Prior to assisted reproduction, regression of endometrial hyperplasia should be achieved as this is associated with higher implantation and clinical pregnancy rates.

HRT and endometrial hyperplasia

- All women taking HRT should be encouraged to report any unscheduled vaginal bleeding promptly.
- There is an increased risk of EH with unopposed oestrogen for 2–3 years.
- Adding in PG reduces its risk.
- Continuous combined HRT is better than sequential PG.
- Stopping sequential HRT can induce regression.
- Women with endometrial hyperplasia taking a sequential HRT preparation who wish to continue HRT should be advised to change to continuous PG intake using the LNG-IUS or a continuous combined HRT preparation.
- Systemic oestrogen-only HRT should not be used in women with a uterus.
- Women with endometrial hyperplasia taking a continuous combined preparation who wish to continue HRT should have their need to continue HRT reviewed.
- Consider using the LNG-IUS as a source of progestogen replacement.

Adjuvant treatment of breast cancer

- Tamoxifen – selective oestrogen receptor modulators (SERM); inhibits proliferation of breast tissue by competitive antagonism of oestrogen receptors
- Partial agonist at other sites – vagina and uterus
- Can promote development of fibroids, polyps and EH
- Increased risk EH with dose and duration
- Aromatase inhibitors – do not increase risk of endometrial pathology/vaginal bleeding

Additional reading

Kurman RJ, Carcangiu ML, Herrington CS, Young RH eds. *WHO Classification of Tumours of Female Reproductive Organs*. 4th ed. Lyon: IARC, 2014.
RCOG/BSGE Joint Guideline. Management of endometrial hyperplasia. *Green-top guideline No. 67*. February 2016. https://www.rcog.org.uk/en/guidelines-research-services/guidelines/gtg67/

15. e

TREATMENT OF VASOMOTOR SYMPTOMS

- Oestrogen and progestogen are given to women with a uterus.
- Oestrogen alone is given to women without a uterus.
- Do not routinely offer SSRIs, serotonin and norepinephrine reuptake inhibitors (SNRIs) or clonidine as first-line treatment for vasomotor symptoms alone.
- Explain to women that there is some evidence that isoflavones or black cohosh may relieve vasomotor symptoms. However, explain that multiple preparations are available and their safety is uncertain.

Women with history of breast cancer

- Offer menopausal women with, or at high risk of, breast cancer: information that the SSRIs paroxetine and fluoxetine should not be offered to women with breast cancer who are taking tamoxifen. (The liver uses the cytochrome P450 enzymes to metabolise many drugs. One of them, CYP2D6, is the principal enzyme that converts tamoxifen into endoxifen, a form that is active in the body. Variations in the gene that synthesises CYP2D6 can limit women's ability to convert tamoxifen into its active form; about 7% of women have no CYP2D6 activity. Some antidepressants that inhibit CYP2D6 enzyme may result in no benefit from tamoxifen. The antidepressants paroxetine, fluoxetine, and bupropion are most likely to inhibit CYP2D6 and interfere with tamoxifen treatment.)

Additional reading

Antidepressants and tamoxifen. Harvard mental health publication. *Harvard Medical School*. http://www.health.harvard.edu/newsletter_article/antidepressants-and-tamoxifen

National Institute for Health and Care Excellence (NICE) *guidance: Menopause diagnosis and management (NG23)*. November 2015. http://www.nice.org.uk/guidance/ng23/chapter/Recommendations#managing-short-term-menopausal-symptoms

PREMATURE OVARIAN FAILURE

Diagnosing premature ovarian insufficiency

- The diagnosis of premature ovarian insufficiency in women aged under 40 years is based on menopausal symptoms, including no or infrequent periods (taking into account whether the woman has a uterus) and elevated FSH levels on two blood samples taken 4–6 weeks apart.
- Do not diagnose premature ovarian insufficiency on the basis of a single blood test.
- Do not routinely use anti-müllerian hormone testing to diagnose premature ovarian insufficiency.
- If there is doubt about the diagnosis of premature ovarian insufficiency, refer the woman to a specialist with expertise in menopause or reproductive medicine.

Managing premature ovarian insufficiency

- Offer sex steroid replacement with a choice of HRT or a combined hormonal contraceptive to women with premature ovarian insufficiency, unless contraindicated (e.g. in women with hormone-sensitive cancer).
- Explain to women with premature ovarian insufficiency the importance of starting hormonal treatment either with HRT or a combined hormonal contraceptive and continuing treatment until at least the age of natural menopause (unless contraindicated).
- Explain that the baseline population risk of diseases such as breast cancer and cardiovascular disease increases with age and is very low in women aged under 40.
- Explain that HRT may have a beneficial effect on blood pressure when compared with a combined oral contraceptive.
- Explain that both HRT and combined oral contraceptives offer bone protection.
- Explain that HRT is not a contraceptive.

Additional reading

National Institute for Health and Care Excellence (NICE) *guidance: Menopause diagnosis and management (NG23)*. November 2015. http://www.nice.org.uk/guidance/ng23/chapter/ Recommendations#managing-short-term-menopausal-symptoms

17. c

UTERINE ARTERY EMBOLISATION (UAE)

Absolute contraindications

- Asymptomatic fibroids
- Recent or current infection of the genital tract
- Pregnancy
- If diagnosis is uncertain due to clinical factors or inadequate imaging
- When patient declines hysterectomy due to social or cultural reasons even after appropriate counselling (small proportion of the patients need hysterectomy following UAE)

Relative contraindications

- Narrow stalk pedunculated submucous fibroid (can get detached and block the cervical canal).
- Large submucous fibroid (may result in sloughing of the fibroid and cause cervical obstruction and occasional sepsis).
- Pedunculated subserosal fibroids (may detach the pedicle and may need laparoscopic removal of these fibroids).
- Evidence not strong enough to absolutely contraindicate UAE in subfertile women. If a woman wants to preserve fertility and has symptomatic fibroids (ovarian failure can occur in 1%–2% although more common in women over 45 years and those who are nearing menopause).

Additional reading

Royal College of Radiologists (RCR) and Royal College of Obstetricians and Gynaecologists (RCOG). *Clinical Recommendations on the Use of Uterine Artery Embolisation (UAE) in the Management of Fibroids.* 3rd ed. 2013. https://www.rcog.org.uk/globalassets/documents/guidelines/23-12-2013_rcog_rcr_uae.pdf

CONTRACEPTION

Questions

1. A 28-year-old, para 2 had a vaginal delivery 20 days ago. She is exclusively breastfeeding her child. She is sexually active but currently not using a contraceptive method. She is hoping that lactation amenorrhoea method (LAM) will prevent her getting pregnant.

   Which one of the following will not increase the risk of her getting pregnant?
   a. Stopping the night feeds
   b. Supplementary feeding
   c. Increase in breastfeeding frequency
   d. Use of pacifiers
   e. Return of menstruation

2. A 28-year-old woman para 4 seeks advice from GP regarding contraception. She had a vaginal delivery 10 days ago but is happy to use the pills.

   Which of the following statements regarding initiating contraception is correct during the postpartum period?
   a. Progesterone-only pill (POP) can be safely started prior to 21 days postpartum.
   b. Use of COC between 6 weeks and 6 months is recommended in fully breastfeeding women
   c. Non-breastfeeding women can start COC before day 21 postpartum
   d. Postpartum women (breastfeeding and non-breastfeeding) can start the POP only after 6 weeks
   e. Breastfeeding women can start COC in the first 6 weeks postpartum as there is sufficient evidence to prove the safety of COC use while establishing breastfeeding

3. **Concerning the use of contraception methods in women with cardiac disease, which one of the following is a correct statement?**
   a. Prophylactic antibiotics are recommended during insertion or removal of intrauterine contraception in women with an increased risk of infective endocarditis
   b. In women on warfarin therapy the risk of bleeding complication is very high during insertion of a progestogen-only implant and therefore its use should be restricted in these women

c. The intrauterine device should be fitted in the hospital setting if the risk of vasovagal reaction is particularly high

d. A causal association has been demonstrated between progestogen-only contraceptive and venous thromboembolism

e. The cardiologist should always be involved in deciding whether to use an intrauterine contraceptive device

4. A 28-year-old woman attends a family planning clinic for contraception advice. She has tested positive for *BRCA1* gene. She has blood pressure (BP) of 140/92 at her last visit with GP.

The following are true regarding contraceptive use for her except which one?

a. She can be advised that there may be an additional risk of breast cancer with COC use

b. She can be advised that there is a reduction in the risk of colorectal cancer with COC use

c. In view of her being a *BRCA1* gene carrier, her risk of ovarian cancer increases by 30% with COC use

d. She can be advised that COC use provides a protective effect against endometrial cancer that continues for 15 years or more after stopping COC

e. Hypertension may increase the risk of stroke and myocardial infarction (MI) in those using COC

5. A 14-year-old girl was having a suction termination of pregnancy (TOP). She did not want her mother to know. Her mother asks you about why her daughter is in the hospital.

The options in the girl's case include the following except for which one?

a. Disclose to the mother

b. Speak to the patient about disclosure

c. Encourage patient to disclose to mother

d. Advise safe sex practices to patient

e. Advise reliable contraception to patient

6. **One of the following conditions does not fall into UKMEC (UK Medical Eligibility Criteria for Contraceptive Use) category 1 for using levonorgestrel intrauterine system (LNG-IUS)**

a. Infections including past pelvic inflammatory disease (PID) with subsequent pregnancy

b. Schistosomiasis (with fibrosis of the liver)

c. Non-pelvic tuberculosis or malaria

d. Infections including past PID without subsequent pregnancy

e. Superficial venous thrombosis (varicose veins or superficial thrombophlebitis)

7. **Which one of the following conditions falls into UKMEC category 3 for using a LNG-IUS?**

a. Complicated valvular and congenital heart disease

b. Women with known pelvic tuberculosis

c. Severe dysmenorrhoea

d. Past history of breast cancer with no recurrence in the last 5 years

e. Undiagnosed breast mass or carriers of gene mutations (e.g. *BRCA1*)

8. A 26-year-old woman para 1 chooses to have a LNG-IUS as a method of contraception. She has been using other forms of contraception.

   In which of the following scenarios mentioned below will this woman need the use of extra protection (condoms or abstinence) for 7 days after insertion?

   a. If the woman is within <12 weeks since last progestogen-only injection

   b. If the woman is within 3 years of insertion of a subdermal implant

   c. If the woman is no later than day 1 of the hormone-free interval for pills or patch

   d. If the woman is within 7 days post-abortion or miscarriage

   e. If the woman is partially breastfeeding, amenorrhoeic and less than 3 months' postpartum

9. **A 20-year-old woman was brought to A&E with a history of sexual assault 4 days ago. The perpetrator had forced her to have vaginal intercourse (used condom) and also performed digital anal penetration. You are the doctor in A&E who is now collecting the samples for forensic medical examination. All the following samples are indicated for forensic medical examination except which one?**

   a. Low vaginal swab

   b. Vulval swab

   c. Peri-anal swab

   d. High vaginal swab

   e. Anal canal swab

10. A 15-year-old girl comes to the family planning clinic for contraception. Her last period was 6 weeks ago and a urine pregnancy test shows a positive result. She expresses a strong wish for termination of pregnancy.

    The following are basic principles for consenting this young person for the procedure except for which one?

    a. A patient can only provide consent if she is deemed to have the capacity to consent to treatment. Gillick competence may be applied

    b. A patient having legal capacity may refuse to have treatment for good/bad reasons or no reason at all and cannot be compelled to have treatment

    c. Competence/capacity in children below the age of 16 years, for instance, teenage pregnant women; the degree of capacity required varies with the seriousness of the decisions to be taken

    d. That the young person understands the procedure and has the maturity to understand what is involved

    e. Consent cannot be revoked by the patient at any time before the treatment is given even if she retains the capacity to do so

11. You are the senior registrar on call for gynaecology. A 15-year-old girl attends emergency department with heavy vaginal bleeding at 16 weeks' gestation and therefore she is taken to theatre for removal of productions of conception

under general anaesthesia. She is haemodynamically unstable and her blood test reveals that the haemoglobin is 5 gm%. The patient is scared and her parents decline to give consent for blood transfusion for their daughter despite explaining that she would die. The parents are Jevohah's Witness. Her partner is at work.

What should the doctor do in this situation?
a. Call the trust solicitor for advice
b. Call the senior sister in charge to talk to the parents
c. Give blood transfusion to save the girl
d. Listen to the parents
e. Wait for her partner to come

1. c

LACTATION AMENORRHOEA METHOD (LAM)

- Women using LAM should be advised that the risk of pregnancy is increased if the frequency of breastfeeding decreases (stopping night feeds, supplementary feeding, use of pacifiers), when menstruation returns or when >6 months postpartum.
- Women may be advised that if they are <6 months postpartum, amenorrhoeic and fully breastfeeding, the LAM method is over 98% effective in preventing pregnancy.
- Women can be informed that available evidence suggests that use of progestogen-only contraception while breastfeeding does not affect breast milk volume.
- Women can be informed that there is currently insufficient evidence to prove whether or not combined oral contraception (COC) affects breast milk volume.
- Women can be informed that progestogen-only contraception has been shown to have no effect on infant growth.

Additional reading

Faculty of sexual and reproductive healthcare clinical guidance – Postnatal sexual and reproductive health (clinical effectiveness unit). September 2009.

2. a
The COC pill should not be started before day 21 postpartum as the risk of thrombosis is high.

Advising women on how and when to start specific contraception methods postpartum Combined oral contraceptive pills

- Women can be advised that contraception is not required before day 21 postpartum. If starting a hormonal method on or before day 21 there is no need for additional contraception.
- If starting a hormonal method after day 21, clinicians should be reasonably sure that the woman is not pregnant or at risk of pregnancy, and should advise that she avoids sex or uses additional contraception for the first 7 days of use (2 days for the POP), unless fully meeting LAM criteria.

- Non-breastfeeding women may start COC from day 21 postpartum.
- Breastfeeding women should avoid COC in the first 6 weeks postpartum as there is insufficient evidence to prove the safety of COC use while establishing breastfeeding.
- Use of COC between 6 weeks and 6 months should not be recommended in fully breastfeeding women unless other methods are not acceptable or available.
- In partially or token breastfeeding women the benefits of COC use may outweigh the risks.

Progesterone-only pills/injectables/implants

- Postpartum women (breastfeeding and non-breastfeeding) can start the POP at any time postpartum.
- Non-breastfeeding women can start a progestogen-only injectable method at any time postpartum.
- Breastfeeding women should not start a progestogen-only injectable method before day 21 unless the risk of subsequent pregnancy is high.
- Women should be advised that troublesome bleeding can occur with use of depot medroxyprogesterone acetate (DMPA) in the early puerperium.
- If more convenient, breastfeeding and non-breastfeeding women can choose to have a progestogen-only implant inserted before day 21, although this is outside the product licence for Implanon.

Intrauterine devices

- Unless a copper-bearing intrauterine device (Cu-IUD) can be inserted within the first 48 hours postpartum (breastfeeding and non-breastfeeding women), insertion should be delayed until day 28 onwards. No additional contraception is required.
- A levonorgestrel-releasing intrauterine system (LNG-IUS) can be inserted from day 28 postpartum (breastfeeding and non-breastfeeding women).
- Women should avoid sex or use additional contraception for 7 days after insertion unless fully meeting LAM criteria.
- Women who choose a diaphragm or cervical cap should be advised to wait at least 6 weeks postpartum before attending for assessment of size requirement.
- Women and men considering sterilisation should be informed of the permanence of the procedure; about the risks, benefits and failure rates associated with sterilisation; and about other methods of contraception including LARC.
- Women can be advised that unprotected sexual intercourse or contraceptive failure before day 21 postpartum is not an indication for emergency contraception.
- Women can be advised that progestogen-only emergency contraception can be used from day 21 onwards and the emergency Cu-IUD from day 28 onwards.

Postpartum contraception choices

Postpartum contraception	Unrestricted	Usually restricted
Not breastfeeding women <21 days postpartum	Barrier methods, POP and injectable progestogen and implants	Any combined hormonal method COCP, vaginal rings and patch IUCD and LGN-IUS unless inserted within 48 hours
Not breastfeeding women >21 days postpartum	COCP POP Progestogen implant and injectables Barrier methods	IUCD and LGN-IUS unless inserted within 48 hours
Breastfeeding women <6 weeks postpartum	Barrier methods POP Progestogen-only implants Lactation amenorrhoea method (LAM)	Any combined hormonal method IUCD and LGN-IUS
Exclusive breastfeeding women from 6 weeks to 6 months	Barrier methods LAM can be used up to 6 months and after this it will be inadequate POP Progestogen injectable and implants IUCD and LGN-IUS	Combined hormonal methods (benefits outweigh risks)
Not exclusively breastfeeding from 6 weeks to 6 months	Barrier methods POP Progestogen injectable and implants IUCD and LGN-IUS	
	Combined hormonal methods (benefits outweigh risks)	
Breastfeeding women >6 months	Barrier methods POP Progestogen-only implants Progestogen injectable and implants IUCD and LGN-IUS	

Additional reading

Faculty of sexual and reproductive healthcare clinical guidance – Postnatal sexual and reproductive health (clinical effectiveness unit). September 2009.
Postpartum contraception. https://patient.info/doctor/postpartum-contraception

3. c

CONTRACEPTION IN WOMEN WITH CARDIAC DISEASE

- Prophylactic antibiotics are not routinely required during insertion or removal of intrauterine contraception in women with an increased risk of infective endocarditis.
- In women on warfarin therapy the risk of bleeding complications is small during insertion of a progestogen-only implant and therefore its use should not be restricted in these women.
- The intrauterine device should be fitted in the hospital setting if the risk of vasovagal reaction is particularly high (e.g. Eisenmenger syndrome, single ventricle, tachycardia or pre-existing bradycardia).
- A causal association has not been demonstrated between progestogen-only contraceptive and venous thromboembolism.
- The use of a combined contraceptive pill is associated with an increased risk of venous thromboembolism.
- A cardiologist should be consulted before deciding whether to use an intrauterine contraceptive device.
- The use of a desogestrel progestogen-only pill may be considered as an interim method while seeking advice about appropriate contraception except for women on enzyme induction medication.

Additional reading

Faculty of sexual and reproductive healthcare clinical guidance – Contraceptive choices for women with cardiac diseases (clinical effectiveness unit). June 2014.

4. c

For women who are at high risk of developing ovarian cancer (such as those who are *BRCA1* and *BRCA2* gene carriers), studies suggest that this risk can be reduced by 60% by using COC pills. Also, a POP may confer an even greater level of protection.

Combined oral contraceptive use risks and benefits

- Women can be advised that CHC use in perimenopause may help to maintain bone mineral density.
- Use of CHC may help to reduce menstrual pain and bleeding.
- Women can be advised that in clinical practice CHC may reduce menopausal symptoms.

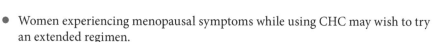

- Women experiencing menopausal symptoms while using CHC may wish to try an extended regimen.
- Women can be advised that there may be a reduction in the incidence of benign breast disease with CHC use.
- Women can be advised that there is a reduction in the risk of colorectal cancer with CHC use.
- Women can be advised that CHC use provides a protective effect against ovarian and endometrial cancer that continues for 15 years or more after stopping CHC.
- Women can be advised that there may be a small additional risk of breast cancer with CHC use, which reduces to no risk 10 years after stopping CHC use.
- Women who are aged 35 years or over and smoke should be advised that the risks of using CHC usually outweigh the benefits.
- Clinicians should be aware that there may be a very small increased risk of ischaemic stroke with CHC use.
- Women with cardiovascular disease, stroke or migraine with aura should be advised against the use of CHC.
- Practitioners who are prescribing CHC to women aged over 40 years may wish to consider a pill with <30 micrograms of ethinylestradiol as a suitable first choice.
- Hypertension may increase the risk of stroke and MI in those using COC.
- Blood pressure should be checked before and at least 6 months after initiating a woman aged over 40 years on CHC and monitored at least annually thereafter.

Additional reading

Faculty of sexual and reproductive healthcare clinical guidance – Contraception for women age over 40 years (clinical effectiveness unit). July 2010.

5. a
Gillick competence or Fraser guidelines: Children under the age of 16 may have the capacity to consent to treatment (if the patient understands information, digests information and is able to make a decision with the information provided), though they cannot refuse treatment. However, they should be encouraged to inform parents but cannot be forced to do so. The information cannot be disclosed to parents unless the patient agrees.

Additional reading

Wheeler R. Gillick or Fraser? A plea for consistency over competence in children: Gillick and Fraser are not interchangeable. *British Medical Journal.* 2006;332(7545):807.

6. d

UKMEC (UK Medical Eligibility Criteria for Contraceptive Use): Definition of categories 1–4
1. A condition for which there is no restriction for the use of the contraceptive method.
2. A condition for which the advantages of using the method generally outweigh the theoretical or proven risks.
3. A condition where the theoretical or proven risks usually outweigh the advantages of using the method.
4. A condition that represents an unacceptable health risk if the contraceptive method is used.
The provision of a method to a woman with a condition given a UKMEC category 3 requires expert clinical judgement and/or referral to a specialist contraceptive provider since use of the method is not usually recommended unless other methods are not available or are not acceptable.

UKMEC for Cu-IUD and the LNG-IUS: UKMEC category 2 (benefits outweigh risks)

- Past PID without subsequent pregnancy
- Continuation of intrauterine methods in women with current PID or purulent cervicitis
- Use in women at increased risk of sexually transmitted infections (STIs) (including HIV, HIV infected or with AIDS and using highly active anti-retroviral therapy [HAART]) or with current infection (excluding HIV and hepatitis) or vaginitis (*Trichomonas vaginalis* or bacterial vaginosis)
- Using HAART
- Anatomic abnormalities not distorting the uterine cavity
- After second-trimester abortion (Ideally intrauterine contraception should be inserted within 48 hours of termination of pregnancy or after 4 weeks; however, exceptions are when other contraceptive methods are unacceptable and the woman wishes to use intrauterine contraception.)
- Continuation of the method in women with cervical cancer awaiting treatment or with endometrial or ovarian cancer

Additional reading

Faculty of sexual and reproductive healthcare clinical guidance – Intrauterine contraception (clinical effectiveness unit). November 2007. http://www.fsrh.org/pdfs/CEUGuidanceintrauterineContraceptionNov07.pdf

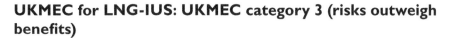

7. d

UKMEC for LNG-IUS: UKMEC category 3 (risks outweigh benefits)

- Continuation of LNG-IUS if a new diagnosis of ischaemic heart disease is made
- If new symptoms of migraine with aura occur at any age
- Past history of breast cancer with no recurrence in last 5 years
- Active viral hepatitis, severely decompensated
- Cirrhosis or liver tumours (benign or malignant)

UKMEC for LNG-IUS: UKMEC category 4 (contraindicated)

- Pregnancy, puerperal sepsis, septic abortion
- Initiation of the method in women with unexplained vaginal bleeding
- Gestational trophoblastic neoplasia when serum hCG concentrations are abnormal
- Initiation of the method in women with cervical cancer awaiting treatment or with endometrial cancer
- Uterine fibroids or uterine anatomical abnormalities distorting the uterine cavity
- Initiation of intrauterine methods in women with current PID or purulent cervicitis
- Initiation of intrauterine methods in women with known pelvic tuberculosis
- Current breast cancer

Additional reading

Faculty of sexual and reproductive healthcare clinical guidance – Intrauterine contraception (clinical effectiveness unit). November 2007. http://www.fsrh.org/pdfs/CEUGuidanceintrauterineContraceptionNov07.pdf

8. e

Note: Following insertion of LNG-IUS, the woman will not need extra protection if her previous contraceptive method is still active.

Timing of Insertion of Cu-IUD/LNG-IUS

A provider can be reasonably certain a woman is not pregnant if she has no symptoms or signs of pregnancy and meets any of the following criteria:

- Has not had intercourse since last normal menses
- Has been correctly and consistently using a reliable method of contraception

- Is within the first 7 days after normal menstrual period.
- Is within the first 7 days post-abortion or miscarriage
- Is fully or nearly fully breastfeeding, amenorrhoeic and less than 6 months' postpartum

Additional reading

Faculty of sexual and reproductive healthcare clinical guidance – Intrauterine contraception (clinical effectiveness unit). November 2007. http://www.fsrh. org/pdfs/CEUGuidanceintrauterineContraceptionNov07.pdf

9. e

Additional reading

Faculty of Forensic and Legal Medicine/Royal College of Paediatric and Child Health (RCPCH). Service specification for the clinical evaluation of children and young people who may have been sexually abused. September 2015. http://www.rcpch.ac.uk/system/files/protected/page/Service%20 Specification%20for%20the%20clinical%20evaluation%20of%20CYP%20 who%20may%20have%20been%20sexually%20abused_September_2015_ FINAL.pdf
Faculty of Forensic and Legal Medicine. Recommendations for the collection of forensic specimens from complainants and suspects. July 2015. http://fflm. ac.uk/wp-content/uploads/2015/10/Recommendations-for-the-collection-of-forensic-specimens-from-july-2015.pdf

10. e

CONSENT

- A proposal of treatment is the first step in obtaining consent and should include a detailed explanation of the nature and purpose of treatment, intended benefits and risks and a discussion of alternatives.
- Concept of 'capacity' or 'competence': All adults (over the age of 18) are presumed to have capacity or competence, and the consent of a child over the age of 16 has the same legal status as that of an adult.

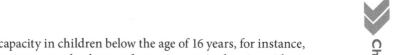

- Competence/capacity in children below the age of 16 years, for instance, teenage pregnant women: the degree of capacity required varies with the seriousness of the decisions to be taken. Fraser guidelines or Gillick competence may be applied (consent for under 16 years of age – that the young person has capacity to consent if she understands the advice and has sufficient maturity to understand what is involved).
- A competent young person under 16 years of age can give consent to medical, surgical and nursing treatment, including contraception and sexual and reproductive health.
- Young people are owed the same duties of care and confidentiality as adults.
- Consent of parents is not legally necessary if Gillick competent.
- Confidentiality may only be broken when the health, safety or welfare of the young person or others would be at grave risk.
- Consent may be revoked at any time before the treatment is given, provided the patient retains the capacity to do so.
- Revocation may be communicated in any form in which consent is communicated.
- Consent is given in advance of treatment and remains valid unless revoked by the patient or circumstances change to remove the basis on which treatment was agreed.

Additional reading

Fraser guidelines or Gillick competence. http://oro.open.ac.uk/15910/1/
Cornock_-_Fraser_guidelines_article.pdf
http://www.fpa.org.uk/factsheets/under-16s-consent-confidentiality
Under 16s: Consent and confidentiality in sexual health services. http://www.fpa.
org.uk/sites/default/files/under-16s-consent-and-confidentiality-factsheet-
march-2009.pdf

11. c
In a life-threatening situation like this, the patient who is under 18 years of age or the parents cannot refuse treatment if it is in the patient's best interest.

General medical council (GMC): 0–18 years guidance:
If a young person refuses treatment

One should respect young people's views in making decisions about their care. If they refuse treatment, particularly treatment that could save their life or prevent serious deterioration in their health, this presents a challenge that you need to consider carefully.

Parents cannot override the competent consent of a young person to treatment that you consider is in their best interests. But you can rely on parental consent when a child lacks the capacity to consent. In Scotland parents cannot authorise treatment a competent young person has refused. In England, Wales and Northern Ireland, the law on parents overriding young people's competent refusal is complex. You should seek legal advice if you think treatment is in the best interests of a competent young person who refuses.

One must carefully weigh the harm to the rights of children and young people of overriding their refusal against the benefits of treatment, so that decisions can be taken in their best interests. In these circumstances, you should consider involving other members of the multi-disciplinary team, an independent advocate, or a named or designated doctor for child protection. Legal advice may be helpful in deciding whether you should apply to the court to resolve disputes about best interests that cannot be resolved informally.

One should also consider involving these same colleagues before seeking legal advice if parents refuse treatment that is clearly in the best interests of a child or young person who lacks capacity, or if both a young person with capacity and their parents refuse such treatment.

Additional reading

Fraser guidelines or Gillick competence. http://oro.open.ac.uk/15910/1/ Cornock_-_Fraser_guidelines_article.pdf http://www.fpa.org.uk/factsheets/ under-16s-consent-confidentiality

GMC guidance on consent. http://www.gmc-uk.org/guidance/ethical_guidance/ children_guidance_30_33_refuse_treatment.asp

Under 16s: Consent and confidentiality in sexual health services. http://www.fpa. org.uk/sites/default/files/under-16s-consent-and-confidentiality-factsheet-march-2009.pdf

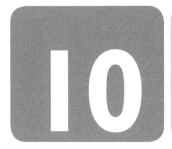

SEXUAL AND REPRODUCTIVE HEALTH

Questions

1. **Gonorrhoea most commonly causes the following except for which one?**
   a. Urethritis
   b. Proctitis
   c. Conjunctivitis
   d. Pharyngitis
   e. Endocarditis

2. **The following facts about chlamydia are true except for which one?**
   a. It is the most common sexually transmitted infection (STI) in the United Kingdom
   b. 3%–7% of sexually active women under 24 years of age have this condition
   c. 70% of women can be asymptomatic
   d. Abnormal menstrual bleeding is not a symptom
   e. If untreated, it can cause sexually acquired reactive arthritis (SARA)

3. **Chlamydia is the most common STI in the United Kingdom. With regards to chlamydia pelvic infection, the following facts are true except for which one?**
   a. It is effectively treated with doxycycline
   b. PID occurs in 10%–15% of untreated women attending GUM with chlamydia
   c. It is treated with erythromycin if diagnosed during pregnancy
   d. Eradication should be checked 4–6 weeks after treatment
   e. Barrier contraception helps to prevent re-infection

4. A 28-year-old woman attends antenatal clinic at 29 weeks of gestation. She recently had visited a sexual health clinic for investigation of her painless vulval ulcer and inguinal lymphadenopathy.

   What treatment would be appropriate for her from the following options?
   a. Benzathine penicillin G single dose as first-line therapy
   b. Azithromycin single dose as first-line therapy
   c. Two doses of benzathine penicillin G to be given 1 week apart
   d. Benzathine penicillin G three weekly doses as first-line therapy
   e. Tetracycline 100 mg three times a day for 14 days

5. A 29-year-old woman attends antenatal clinic at 28 weeks of gestation. She gives a history of syphilis 2 years ago. She has recently been diagnosed with late syphilis and now advised to have a cerebrospinal fluid (CSF) examination test.

The indications for CSF examination include all of the following except for which one?
a. Ophthalmic signs and symptoms
b. Syphilis treatment failure
c. Neurological signs and symptoms
d. Cardiovascular signs and symptoms
e. HIV infection with late latent syphilis

6. A 25-year-old woman presents to A&E with painful vulva. Examination reveals multiple ulcers (around the fourchette) with ragged undermined edges with necrotic base and purulent exudate. There was contact bleeding. Also noted were enlarged tender left inguinal lymph modes.

The like diagnosis in her case is which of the following?
a. Lymphogranuloma venerum
b. Syphillis gummata
c. Chancroid
d. Donovanosis
e. Type 2 herpes simplex infection

7. A 23-year-old woman presents to the sexual health clinic with warty lesions on her vulva. Examination reveals warts on the vulva and the lower part of vagina but not obstructing the vagina. She is currently 16 weeks by dates and is booked for an anomaly scan at 20 weeks.

How would you treat her at this stage?
a. Podophylline
b. Trichloroacetic acid
c. 5-Fluorouracil
d. Excision of all lesions under general anaesthesia
e. Interferons

8. A 66-year-old woman is referred to the vulval clinic as a 2-week wait. She is para 2 with premature menopause. She has been taking hormone replacement therapy (HRT) for the last 27 years. She gives history of vulval itching, soreness and superficial dyspareunia. Clinical examination reveals erythematous changes within the vulval skin with fissuring, excoriation and oedema. Satellite lesions are seen on the inner thigh and lower abdomen.

A probable diagnosis in her case is which of the following?
a. Lichen sclerosis
b. Lichen planus
c. Candidiasis
d. Donovanosis
e. Lichen simplex

9. A 35-year-old woman presented with a frothy vaginal discharge that is fishy in odour. On speculum examination, the cervix was red, punctate and inflamed. The wet mount shows the mobile organism.

What is a likely diagnosis in her case?
a. Trichomoniasis
b. Candidiasis
c. Bacterial vaginosis
d. Chlamydia
e. Donovanosis

10. A woman who is 14 weeks pregnant presents with a thin vaginal discharge and fishy odour. She gives history of this getting worse before her periods and with sexual intercourse. On examination, the vulva and vagina looked normal and not inflamed.

The diagnosis in her case is which of the following?
a. Tricomoniasis
b. Candidiasis
c. Bacterial vaginosis
d. Chlamydia
e. Donovanosis

11. A 20-year-old woman attends the sexual health clinic with symptoms of frothy, yellow vaginal discharge and associated lower abdominal pain. The organism can be seen when a drop of saline is added to the vaginal discharge placed on the slide.

What is the most likely diagnosis?
a. Chlamydia
b. *Trichomonas vaginalis*
c. Gonorrhoea
d. *Candida albicans*
e. Syphilis

12. A 16-year-old woman attends the sexual health clinic with a complaint of thin homogenous vaginal discharge for 2 weeks. A vaginal wet mount smear shows clue cells.

What is the most likely diagnosis?
a. *Treponema pallidum*
b. ß-Haemolytic streptococci
c. *Gardnerella vaginalis*
d. Herpes simplex
e. Donovanosis

Answers

1. e

Gram-negative diplococcus is the causative organism for gonorrhoea. It usually infects mucous membranes (endocervix, pharynx, rectum, urethra and conjunctiva). It also facilitates HIV transmission. Women present with abnormal vaginal discharge (short incubation period: 3–5 days). In 50% of women there are no symptoms.

The diagnosis is confirmed by detection of the organism by Gram staining of the vaginal discharge (reveals gram-negative diplococci) in the first few days following infection. It facilitates transmission of HIV. Endocervical swabs can be taken for nucleic acid amplification techniques (NAATs). Generally, the antibiotic of choice is ceftriaxone 500 mg intramuscular (IM) stat dose though this may vary as per organism sensitivity and local hospital protocol. One should also treat the patient for chlamydia. Contact tracing and treatment of partners is very important to prevent recurrences.

Additional reading

Lazaro, N. *Sexually Transmitted Infections in Primary Care.* 2nd ed. RCGP/ BASHH. 2013. www.bashh.org/documents/Sexually%20Transmitted%20 Infections%20in%20Primary%20Care%202013.pdf

2. d

CHLAMYDIA

Chlamydia is caused by obligate intracellular pathogen which usually affects the mucous membranes of the endocervix, rectum, urethra, conjunctiva and pharynx. The risk factors include below the age of 25 years, recent sexual partner, more than one partner within the previous year and lack of consistent use of condoms. Women can present with vaginal discharge, dysuria, lower abdominal pain, deep dyspareunia, cervicitis, postcoital bleeding and intermenstrual bleeding. Oedematous cervix and contact bleeding (cervix) can be seen on speculum examination. For diagnosis, an endocervical swab is needed for culture or for NAAT to identify DNA.

If not treated, chlamydia may cause severe complications which include pelvic inflammatory disease (PID) (without treatment 10%–40% will develop PID), infertility, chronic pelvic pain, adult conjunctivitis, neonatal conjunctivitis (30%– 50% may develop infection of eyes, nasopharynx, genitalia and lungs), SARA, perihepatitis (Fitz-Hugh and Curtis syndrome), preterm delivery, increase risk of

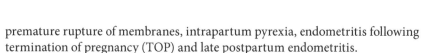

premature rupture of membranes, intrapartum pyrexia, endometritis following termination of pregnancy (TOP) and late postpartum endometritis.

A referral to a genito-urinary medicine (GUM) clinic is necessary for full screen of STIs and should include treatment of the partner. Chlamydia is treated with doxycycline (100 mg orally twice daily for 14 days) or azithromycin 1 gm stat dose orally (if compliance is the issue). During pregnancy erythromycin should be used as doxycycline is contraindicated.

Additional reading

Lazaro, N. *Sexually Transmitted Infections in Primary Care.* 2nd ed. RCGP/ BASHH. 2013. www.bashh.org/documents/Sexually%20Transmitted%20 Infections%20in%20Primary%20Care%202013.pdf

3. e

FACTS ABOUT CHLAMYDIA INFECTION IN THE UNITED KINGDOM

Women below the age of 25 years, recent sexual partner, more than one partner within the previous year and lack of consistent use of condoms are risk factors. Barrier contraceptives are likely to protect against STIs that are usually transmitted by genital fluids such as chlamydia, gonorrhoea, trichomoniasis and HIV infection. They are unlikely to protect from diseases that are transmitted by skin-to-skin contact.

In the United Kingdom, 3%–7% (6%) of sexually active women under 24 years of age have this condition. About 50%–70% of women can be asymptomatic. In the United Kingdom, chlamydia is detected in 10% of women requesting TOP. If not treated it will result in acute and chronic sequelae which include acute PID, pelvic pain, infertility (5%–18%), ectopic pregnancy and psychological problems. If detected prior to TOP and not treated 20%–25% of these women will develop post-abortal pelvic infection and its sequelae.

Additional reading

Centers for Disease Control and Prevention (CDC). https://www.cdc.gov/ condomeffectiveness/brief.html

Lazaro, N. *Sexually Transmitted Infections in Primary Care.* 2nd ed. RCGP/ BASHH. 2013. www.bashh.org/documents/Sexually%20Transmitted%20 Infections%20in%20Primary%20Care%202013.pdf

4. c

(In her case the diagnosis is early syphilis.)

MANAGEMENT OF SYPHILIS DURING PREGNANCY

- **Early syphilis:** First and second trimesters: give benzathine penicillin G, single dose. In third trimester, a second dose of benzathine penicillin G to be given 1 week after the first. Ceftriaxone 500 mg IM ×10 days added to alternatives.
- **Late syphilis:** Benzathine penicillin G three weekly doses first-line therapy (except for neurosyphilis: procaine penicillin G with concomitant oral probenecid remains first-line therapy for this).
- **HIV-positive patients**: Treat as appropriate for the stage of infection as HIV-positive patients are treated with the same regimes as HIV-negative patients.
- During pregnancy, a referral to a foetal medicine consultant for evaluation of foetal effects during treatment is recommended after 26 weeks' gestation.

Additional reading

British Association for Sexual Health and HIV (Clinical Effectiveness Group): UK National Guidelines on the Management of Syphilis 2008. https://stratog. rcog.org.uk/files/rcog-corp/elearn/38687/48858/bashh_syphilis.pdf

5. d

INDICATIONS FOR CSF EXAMINATION IN LATE SYPHILIS INFECTION INCLUDE

- Ophthalmic signs and symptoms
- Syphilis treatment failure
- Neurological signs and symptoms
- HIV infection with late latent syphilis or syphilis with unknown duration

Interpretation of CSF serology should be done carefully

- CSF should not be macroscopically contaminated with blood.
- Positive syphilis tests on CSF should be interpreted in conjunction with biochemical examination of the CSF as well as clinical signs and symptoms.
- Most people with symptomatic neurosyphilis have a raised white cell count in the CSF (>5 cells/mm^3).

- Positive CSF VDRL (venereal disease research laboratory) and CSF TPPA (*Treponema pallidum* particle agglutination assay) tests should be repeated quantitatively. The overall sensitivity of the CSF VDRL/RPR (rapid plasma reagin) is around 50% with a range of 10% for asymptomatic cases to 90% for symptomatic cases.
- A negative CSF VDRL/RPR does not exclude neurosyphilis though a positive CSF VDRL/RPR (in the absence of substantial contamination of CSF with blood) is diagnostic of neurosyphilis.
- A negative treponemal test on CSF excludes neurosyphilis. A positive test is highly sensitive for neurosyphilis but lacks specificity because reactivity may be caused by transudation of immunoglobulins from the serum into the CSF or by leakage through a damaged blood-brain barrier resulting from conditions other than syphilis.
- Neurosyphilis is unlikely when the CSF TPHA (fluorescent treponemal antibody absorption [FTA-ABS]) titre is <320 and a CSF TPPA titre <640.
- A TPHA index >70 and a CSF TPHA titre >320 are the most reliable indices in supporting a diagnosis of neurosyphilis but unfortunately determination of the TPHA index is not widely available.

Additional reading

British Association for Sexual Health and HIV (Clinical Effectiveness Group). UK National Guidelines on the Management of Syphilis 2008. https://stratog. rcog.org.uk/files/rcog-corp/elearn/38687/48858/bashh_syphilis.pdf

CDC STD treatment guidelines 2002. *MMWR*. 2002;51(RR-6).

6. c

CHANCROID

Chancroid, caused by infection with *Haemophilus ducreyi*, presents with anogenital ulceration plus lymphadenitis and the formation of bubo (abscess). This is found in 50% of cases and is mostly unilateral. Buboes form and can become fluctuant and rupture, releasing thick pus, resulting sometimes in extensive ulceration. The incubation period ranges between 3 and 10 days.

Diagnosis

Culture from the ulcer base, or the undermined edges of the ulcer or from pus aspirated from the bubo should be obtained. This is then transferred on to culture media (incubated at 33°C in high humidity with 5% carbon dioxide for a minimum of 48–72 hours).

Treatment of chancroid

- Single-dose oral azithromycin (1 g) or ciprofloxacin (500 mg), which are effective in 90%–95% of cases.
- Azithromycin 1 g orally in a single dose (Ib, grading A) or
- Ceftriaxone 250 mg intramuscularly (IM) in a single dose (Ib, B) or
- Ciprofloxacin 500 mg orally in a single dose (Ib, B) or
- Ciprofloxacin 500 mg orally two times a day for 3 days (Ib, B/A) or
- Erythromycin base 500 mg orally four times a day for 7 days (Ib, B/A)

Note regarding allergy: Patients allergic to quinolones or cephalosporins should be treated with the erythromycin regimen.

Grades of recommendations

Code	Quality of evidence	Definition
A	High	Further research is very unlikely to change our confidence in the estimate of effect. At least one meta-analysis, systematic review or randomised controlled trial (RCT)
B	Moderate	Further research is likely to have an important impact on our confidence in the estimate of effect and may change the estimate One high-quality study Several studies with some limitations
C	Low	Further research is very likely to have an important impact on our confidence in the estimate of effect and is likely to change the estimate One or more studies with severe limitations
D	Very low	Any estimate of effect is very uncertain Expert opinion No direct research evidence

Ulcers heal within a few days of treatment. However, patients should be advised to avoid unprotected sexual intercourse until they and their partner(s) have completed treatment and follow-up. Investigations for other possible causes of genital ulcerative disease should be performed (especially for *Treponema pallidum* and genital herpes), and also if necessary for lymphogranuloma venereum (LGV) or donovanosis. Testing for HIV should be considered.

Treatment for pregnant or lactating mothers and children

- The safety of azithromycin for pregnant and lactating women is uncertain.
- Ciprofloxacin is contraindicated for pregnant and lactating women, children, and adolescents less than 18 years of age.
- The erythromycin or ceftriaxone regimens can be used.
- No adverse effects of chancroid on pregnancy outcome or on the foetus have been reported.

Follow-up

- Patients should be re-examined 3–7 days after initiation of therapy.
- If treatment is successful, ulcers improve symptomatically within 3 days and substantial re- epithelization occurs within 7 days after onset of therapy.
- The time required for complete healing is related to the size of the ulcer (and perhaps HIV-related immunosuppression); large ulcers may require more than 2 weeks to heal.

Additional reading

BASSH guidelines. Management of chancroid. 2007. https://stratog.rcog.org.uk/files/rcog-corp/elearn/38687/48883/chancroid_2007.pdf

Clinical governance advice No 1c. Development of RCOG green top guideline: Producing a clinical practice guideline. Revised. November 2006. https://www.rcog.org.uk/globalassets/documents/guidelines/clinical-governance-advice/clinical-governance-advice-1c.pdf

Levels of evidence. https://www.essentialevidenceplus.com/product/ebm_loe.cfm?show=grade

7. b

ANOGENITAL WARTS

Anogenital warts are caused by the human papillomavirus (HPV) (over 100 genotypes have been identified). The mode of transmission is most often by sexual contact but HPV may be transmitted perinatally and genital lesions resulting from transfer of infection from hand warts have been reported in children. There is no good evidence of transmission from fomites. Mostly they are caused by HPV types 6 and 11.

- Extragenital lesions may be seen on the oral cavity, larynx, conjunctivae and nasal cavity.

Clinical appearances of exophytic warts

- Warts may be single or multiple.
- Those on the warm, moist, non-hair-bearing skin tend to be soft and non-keratinised and those on the dry hairy skin firm and keratinised.
- Lesions may be broad based or pedunculated and some are pigmented.

Treatment options of anogenital warts

- The topical use of podophyllin paint on the vulval and perianal warts
- Trichloroacetic acid (TCA) on vaginal and cervical warts
- Cryotherapy with liquid nitrogen is widely used.
- Diathermy, laser treatment and excision of more extensive genital warts under local or even general anaesthetic may be considered in more severe or resistant cases.
- Immuno-modifying agents, such as imiquimod, and interferons may be considered for these patients.
- Topical therapy with 5-fluorouracil (5-FU) is now only considered rarely.
- Soft non-keratinised warts respond well to podophyllin, podophyllotoxin and trichloroacetic acid.
- Keratinised lesions are better treated with physical ablative methods such as cryotherapy, excision or electrocautery.
- Imiquimod may be suitable for both keratinised and non-keratinised warts.
- People with fewer and low volume warts are best treated with ablative therapy from the outset.
- Podophyllotoxin, for 4-week cycles, and imiquimod for up to 16 weeks are suitable for home treatment by patients. If chosen, the patient should be given a demonstration on lesion finding and treatment application.
- Local anaesthetic creams plus or minus injection with an injectable local anaesthetic (e.g. 2% lignocaine) could be used before ablative therapy to minimise discomfort. Adrenaline-containing anaesthetic should be avoided for lesions on the penis and around the clitoris.
- No treatment is an option at any site and may apply particularly to warts in the vagina and anal canal as they should regress in time.

Treatment of anogenital warts during pregnancy

The options for the treatment of anogenital warts during pregnancy are limited by potential teratogenicity of some modalities such as podophyllin. TCA and imiquimod can be used safely, as well as ablative techniques, such as cryotherapy. Treatment of the warts may reduce transmission of the HPV to the foetus during vaginal delivery.

Additional reading

BASSH guidelines. Management of anogenital warts. 2007. https://stratog.rcog.org. uk/files/rcog-corp/elearn/38687/48747/bashh_warts.pdf

CANDIDIASIS

Risk factors

- Uncontrolled diabetes mellitus
- Immunosuppression
- Hyperoestrogenaemia (including HRT and the combined oral contraceptive pill)
- Use of broad-spectrum antibiotics (causes disturbance of vaginal flora)

Presentation of candidiasis

- Vulval itching
- Soreness
- Vaginal discharge
- Superficial dyspareunia
- External dysuria

Signs on examination of vulva and vagina

- Erythematous change within the vulval skin
- Fissuring, excoriation and oedema
- Satellite lesions may occur on the inner thigh and lower abdomen
- The vaginal discharge may be 'curdy', having the appearance of small pieces of milk curd or cottage cheese–like material within a pale gray or white discharge
- Discharge is non-offensive

Diagnosis of candidiasis

High vaginal swab and culture. A diagnosis is made if pseudohyphae or yeast buds are present. (These are visible only 50% of the time.)

Types of candidiasis classified for treatment purpose

- Uncomplicated candidiasis
- Complicated candidiasis

Management of uncomplicated vulvovaginal candidiasis

Topical and oral azole therapies are used (achieve a clinical and mycological cure rate of over 80%).

Management of complicated vulvovaginal candidiasis

Vulvovaginal candidiasis is regarded as complicated when one of the following are present

- Severe symptoms.
- Pregnancy: Topical imidazoles should be used for symptomatic vulvovaginal candidiasis in pregnancy. Longer courses are recommended; a 4-day course will cure just over 50%, whereas a 7-day course cures over 90%. Oral therapy is contraindicated.
- Recurrent vulvovaginal candidiasis (more than four symptomatic attacks per year). A positive microscopy or a moderate/heavy growth of *Candida albicans* should be documented on at least two occasions when symptomatic. (Approximately 5% of women of reproductive age with a primary episode of vulvovaginal candidiasis will develop recurrent disease.)
- Non-albicans species.
- Abnormal host (e.g. hyper-oestrogenic state, diabetes mellitus, immunosuppression).

Treatment is based on two principles: Induction and maintenance therapy

Induction dose: Fluconazole 150 mg every 3 days for three doses
Maintenance dose: Fluconazole 150 mg every week for 6 months

Alternative regimen

Induction therapy: Topical imidazole therapy can be increased to 10–14 days according to symptomatic response.
Maintenance therapy: Fluconazole 50 mg daily or clotrimazole 500 mg once a week vaginal pessary.

Note

- Fluconazole is contraindicated during pregnancy and breastfeeding.
- If relapse occur between doses, one should consider twice-weekly 150 mg fluconazole or 50 mg fluconazole daily.
- If there is an underlying dermatitis then she may need a steroid cream or a combination of antifungal and steroid cream. An emollient is also necessary.

Additional reading

StratOG: The RCOGs online learning source. https://stratog.rcog.org.uk/tutorial/
sexually-transmitted-infections-including-hiv/candidal-infection-3822
UK National Guideline on the Management of Vulvovaginal Candidiasis. 2007.
http://www.bashh.org/documents/1798.pdf

TRICHOMONAS VAGINALIS

- Urethral infection is present in 90% of cases.
- It is a sexually transmitted condition.
- Approximately 50% of infected women are asymptomatic.
- The most common symptoms include vaginal discharge (vaginits), vulval itching (vulvitis), dysuria or an offensive odour.
- There may occasionally be lower abdominal pain.
- Vaginal discharge is present in 70% of cases – classical frothy, yellow-green discharge and bad smelling.
- The so-called 'strawberry cervix' with its characteristic vascular pattern is only present in 2% of cases, although this may be more visible at colposcopy.
- Diagnosis rests on direct observation of the organism on a wet smear (mobile trichomonads are visible on the slide).
- Specialised culture media are required and will be diagnostic in 95% of cases.
- Trichomonads may occasionally be seen on cervical smears, though not all laboratories will report them because of a significant false-positive rate. It is prudent to confirm the diagnosis by direct observation or culture.

Additional reading

BASSH guidelines. Management of *Tricomonas vaginalis*. 2007. https://stratog. rcog.org.uk/tutorial/sexually-transmitted-infections-including-hiv/ trichomonas-infection-3817

10. c

BACTERIAL VAGINOSIS (BV)

Bacterial vaginosis generally produces a vaginal discharge that is thin and milky with a fishy odour. Symptoms and signs include fishy, offensive, thin watery discharge without any associated itch or inflammation. A vaginal wet mount shows clue cells. Around 50%–75% of women who have BV do not have any symptoms but those who do often complain of a fishy smelling vaginal odour and a milky-white, or grey vaginal discharge. The odour may get worse around the time of menstruation or after unprotected sexual intercourse. When semen (male sperm) mixes with vaginal secretions, the odour becomes stronger. Less common symptoms include vaginal itchiness, redness and pain with intercourse.

Diagnosis is made if >20% of cells are clue cells (and two of the following three criteria are met).

Amsel's Criteria:

- Discharge is thin and homogeneous.
- Sample smells fishy when mixed with potassium hydroxide (whiff test).
- Vaginal pH is >4.5. (Vaginal pH test: Normal vaginal pH is 3.8–4.5. Bacterial vaginosis, trichomoniasis and atrophic vaginitis often cause a vaginal pH higher than 4.5.)

Additional reading

FFPRHC (Faculty of Family Planning and Reproductive Health Care) and BASHH Guidance. The management of women of reproductive age attending non-genitourinary medicine settings complaining of vaginal discharge. *Journal of Family Planning and Reproductive Health Care*. 2006;32(1):33–42.

StratOG: The ROCGs online learning source. https://stratog.rcog.org.uk/files/rcog-corp/elearn/38687/48901/vaginaldischargeguidance.pdf

11. b

Additional reading

BASSH guidelines. Management of *Tricomonas vaginalis*. 2007. https://stratog.rcog.org.uk/tutorial/sexually-transmitted-infections-including-hiv/trichomonas-infection-3817

12. c

Additional reading

FFPRHC (Faculty of Family Planning and Reproductive Health Care) and BASHH Guidance. The management of women of reproductive age attending non-genitourinary medicine settings complaining of vaginal discharge. *Journal of Family Planning and Reproductive Health Care*. 2006;32(1):33–42.

StratOG: The ROCGs online learning source. https://stratog.rcog.org.uk/tutorial/sexually-transmitted-infections-including-hiv

GENETIC PROBLEMS

Questions

1. A 28-year-old woman is referred to the geneticist for counselling. Her son died at 6 years of age in Pakistan but had not been tested for any genetic condition. She was told it was a congenital condition.

   For her future pregnancies pre-implantation genetic testing can be offered to detect the following, except which one condition?
   a. Cystic fibrosis
   b. Foetal sex
   c. Duchenne muscular dystrophy
   d. Spinal muscular atrophy type 1
   e. Down syndrome

2. A 45-year-old women gravid 1 para 0 is referred to antenatal clinic for booking. She misses her dating scan. She is now 16 weeks' pregnant and her booking bloods reveal normal haematological and biochemical tests. However, her quadruple test reveals low levels of AFP (α-fetoprotein) and oestriol and high levels of ß-hCG and inhibin A. Karyotyping report following amniocentesis is reported as 47XX,+21.

   The associated risks to the foetus include all except which one of the following?
   a. Hirschsprung disease
   b. Congenital heart disease
   c. Acute leukaemia
   d. Low IQ of 25–50
   e. Spina bifida

3. A 43-year-old woman gravid 1 para 0 is referred to the antenatal clinic for booking. Her dating scan at 13 weeks shows increased nuchal thickness. Chorionic villus sampling (CVS) results show trisomy 21.

   Which one of the following is not associated with Down syndrome?
   a. Clinodactyly of the little finger (fifth finger)
   b. Congenital deafness
   c. Non-disjunction
   d. Single palmar crease
   e. Atrial septal defect

4. A 35-year-old woman presents to the early pregnancy unit with moderate vaginal bleeding. An ultrasound is performed, which reports a complete molar pregnancy.

   What would be the genetic complement and parental origin of the complete molar pregnancy?
   a. Haploid: two paternal sets
   b. Diploid: two paternal sets
   c. Triploid: paternal and maternal
   d. Tetraploid: two paternal and two maternal set
   e. Diploid: one maternal and one paternal set

5. **Genetic syndromes are associated with different gene mutations. The following are correctly matched except which one?**
   a. Cowden syndrome: Germline *PTEN* mutations
   b. Hereditary breast and ovarian cancer *BRCA1/BRCA2*
   c. Lynch syndrome: *MSH6*
   d. Li-Fraumeni syndrome: Germline *TP53* mutations
   e. Peutz-Jeghers syndrome: *PMS2*

6. **What is the most likely chromosomal abnormality responsible for truncus arteriosus?**
   a. Trisomy 13
   b. Trisomy 21
   c. Chromosome 22q11 deletions
   d. 46 XXY syndrome
   e. Trisomy 18

7. A 29-year-old woman is planning to conceive. Her brother is diagnosed with haemophilia A.

   The following offspring in her family are at risk of developing haemophilia in the scenarios described below except for which one?
   a. A female child whose mother is a carrier and has an affected father with haemophilia
   b. A male child of a healthy female silently carrying the faulty gene
   c. A male child whose father has the deficient gene
   d. A female child with Turner syndrome whose mother is carrying the deficient gene
   e. A male child with an affected cousin on his mother's side

8. **Which one of the following statements is true regarding foetal isoimmune erythroblastic anaemia?**
   a. Mirror syndrome is associated with maternal anaemia
   b. Doppler artery waveforms in the uterine artery predict foetal anaemia
   c. Anti-D levels are considered significant only above 60 IU/mL
   d. Repeated amniocentesis does not help in reliable monitoring of anti-Kell disease
   e. Middle cerebral artery Doppler waveforms accurately predict foetal anaemia

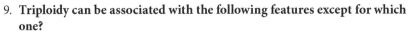

9. **Triploidy can be associated with the following features except for which one?**
   a. Partial hydatidiform mole
   b. Severe intrauterine growth restriction
   c. First-trimester spontaneous abortions
   d. Three sets of diploid chromosomes
   e. Fertilisation of diploid sperm

10. **The following conditions are transmitted as autosomal dominant except for which one?**
    a. Hereditary spherocytosis
    b. Von Hippel-Lindau syndrome
    c. Tuberous sclerosis
    d. Xeroderma pigmentosum
    e. Neurofibromatosis (von Recklinghausen disease)

11. **The following genetic conditions except one, only manifest when an individual is homozygous and heterozygous for the mutant allele. Which condition is the exception?**
    a. Adult polycystic kidney disease
    b. Familial adenomatous polyposis coli
    c. Fanconi anaemia
    d. Gilbert syndrome
    e. Huntington chorea

12. **The following conditions except one manifest only when the individual is homozygous for the mutant allele. Which one is the exception?**
    a. Galactosaemia
    b. G6PD deficiency
    c. Glycogen storage diseases
    d. Homocystinuria
    e. Marfan syndrome

Answers

1. **c**

PRE-IMPLANTATION GENETIC DIAGNOSIS (PGD)

Pre-implantation genetic diagnosis (PGD) is a technique that involves testing the embryo after *in vitro* fertilisation in women with a specific inherited condition in their family to avoid transferring it to their children. One or two cells (blastomeres) are aspirated from the pre-implantation embryo on day 3 of development (6–10 cell stage). Following this procedure, unaffected embryos are transferred into the uterus.

Uses of PGD

- It can be used to determine the foetal sex to identify sex-linked disorders.
- It can be used to detect various chromosomal abnormalities. Fluorescence in situ hybridisation (FISH) has to be used to detect these chromosomal re-arrangements which include chromosome deletions, inversions and translocations.
- It can be used to detect single gene defects (e.g. cystic fibrosis). The molecular abnormality is tested with techniques after polymerase chain reaction (PCR) of the DNA extracted from single cells.

The list of conditions for which PGD can be offered (licensed) is published by HFEA (Human Fertilisation and Embryology Authority).

Additional reading

Human Fertilisation and Embryology Authority (HFEA). Preimplantation genetic diagnosis. https://www.hfea.gov.uk/treatments/embryo-testing-and-treatments-for-disease/pre-implantation-genetic-diagnosis-pgd/

2. **e**

In this case the foetus has Down syndrome (trisomy 21). This is a condition which results from non-disjunction (95% of cases) or chromosomal translocation (5% of cases). The incidence is 1 in 700 live births. The incidence increases with increasing maternal age.

Quadruple screen test

It is a test performed during pregnancy (between 16 and 18 weeks) to determine whether the baby is at risk of developing certain congenial birth defects or genetic abnormalities.

The following hormonal blood tests are included in the quadruple test:

- AFP – produced by the baby
- ß-hCG – produced in the placenta
- Unconjugated oestriol (uE3) – produced in the foetus and placenta
- Inhibin A – released by the placenta

AFP is a glycoprotein which is produced in the foetal liver, yolk sac and gastrointestinal tract. Maternal serum AFP rises from 10 to 32 weeks of gestation and declines thereafter. Foetal serum concentration rises from the fourth week and peaks at 12–14 weeks of gestation. Serum AFP falls progressively towards the term or 37 weeks of pregnancy.

High levels of maternal serum AFP is seen in the following conditions

- Anencephaly
- Duodenal atresia
- Spina bifida
- Tetralogy of Fallot
- Intrauterine death of foetus
- Multiple gestation
- Abdominal wall defects (exomphalos)
- Error in dates
- Methylenetetradydrofolate reductase genetic variant in mother
- Ovarian germ cell tumour in the mother

Low levels of maternal serum AFP is seen in the following conditions

- Trisomy 21
- Trisomy 18
- Diabetes mellitus in mother

Additional reading

Collins S et al. *Oxford Handbook of Obstetrics and Gynaecology.* 3rd ed. Oxford: Oxford University Press; 2013.

3. b

Down syndrome is the most common chromosomal abnormality in newborn babies. The incidence of this condition is related to maternal age. The majority (95%) occur due to non-disjunction and 5% are due to chromosomal translocations (inherited from a parent with balanced chromosomal translocation carrier).

The main diagnostic tests used to diagnose Down syndrome include CVS, amniocentesis and free foetal DNA in maternal blood.

Chorionic villus biopsy is usually performed from 11 weeks of gestation. The results are available earlier than with amniocentesis. The miscarriage rate is 2%.

Amniocentesis is usually performed at 15–16 weeks of gestation. The risks associated with this procedure include culture failure (0.5%), miscarriage (0.5%–1%) and delay in obtaining the results (may be reduced by the use of FISH in situ hybridisation technique).

Additional reading

Collins S et al. *Oxford Handbook of Obstetrics and Gynaecology*. 3rd ed. Oxford: Oxford University Press; 2013.

4. b

In most cases of complete molar pregnancy, all the genetic material is inherited from the father. In approximately 80% of these, a possible mechanism is that a single sperm fertilises an empty egg followed by a duplication of all of the chromosomes. In the rest of the cases (20%) an empty egg is fertilised by two sperms. In both cases, the molar pregnancies are diploid.

Additional reading

Gestational trophoblastic disease. Green-top guideline No 38. 2010. https://www.rcog.org.uk/womens-health/clinical-guidance/management-gestational-trophoblastic-neoplasia-green-top-38
Hoffner L, Surti U. The genetics of gestational trophoblastic disease: A rare complication of pregnancy. *Cancer Genetics*. 2012;205(3):63–77.

COWDEN SYNDROME

- Germline mutations in tumour suppressor gene *PTEN*
- Autosomal dominant condition presenting in adulthood
- Endometrial cancer is one of the major diagnostic criteria (lifetime risk 30%)
- Hamartomatous bowel polyps, skin and mucosal lesions
- Benign and malignant tumours of breast and thyroid
- Also associated with melanoma, colorectal and renal cell carcinomas
- Macrocephaly >98th centile
- Developmental delay: Bannayan-Riley-Ruvalcaba syndrome in children

Risk-reducing hysterectomy may be discussed with these women although data on efficacy are limited.

Peutz-Jeghers Syndrome

- Germline mutations in the *STK11* gene
- Autosomal dominant condition
- Gastrointestinal polyposis disorder
- Characteristic pigmented lesions on the lips and buccal mucosa
- Increased risk of breast, gastrointestinal and gynaecological tumours
- Increased risk of sex cord stromal tumours with annular tubules of the ovary and adenoma malignum of the cervix
- Annual Pap smear from the age 18 years and TVS and Ca125 measurements from 25 years are suggested

Li-Fraumeni syndrome (LFS)

- Germline *TP53* mutations
- Young-onset sarcomas, breast cancer, adrenocortical carcinoma and childhood tumours
- Gynaecological cancers are unusual in LFS, the most common one being epithelial ovarian carcinoma

Lynch syndrome

- Associated with *MLH1*, *MSH2*, *MSH6*, *PMS2* genes

Additional reading

Royal College of Obstetricians and Gynaecologists (RCOG). Management of women with genetic predisposition to gynaecological cancers. Scientific impact paper No 48. February 2015.

6. c

TRUNCUS ARTERIOSUS

This is caused because of incomplete or failed septation of the embryonic truncus arteriosus. Mostly it occurs spontaneously but can also be caused by chromosomal abnormalities and teratogens. In 40%–50% of the cases, the associated chromosomal abnormality is chromosome 22q11 deletions (DiGeorge Syndrome). The other features of chromosome 22q11 deletions include cardiac abnormality especially tetralogy of Fallot, abnormal facies, thymic aplasia, cleft palate, hypocalcemia, hypoparathyroidism and learning disability.

The anatomical changes include single artery arising from the two ventricles which give rise to both aortic and pulmonary vessels, right-sided aortic arch, abnormal truncal valve, large ventricular septal defect (VSD), pulmonary hypertension, right-to-left shunt and complete mixing of blood occurring at the level of the great vessels.

Additional reading

Available at: http://emedicine.medscape.com/article/892489-overview
Collins S et al. *Oxford Handbook of Obstetrics and Gynaecology*. 3rd ed. Oxford: Oxford University Press; 2013.

7. c

HAEMOPHILIA A

- This is an X (Sex)-linked recessive condition.
- It is more likely to occur in males than in females.
- Females are almost exclusively asymptomatic carriers.
- Female carriers pass the defective X chromosome to 50% of the sons.
- If the mother is affected with haemophilia, the defective gene is passed to 100% of the sons.
- For a female to inherit the disease, she must receive two deficient X chromosomes (one from father and one from mother). If the father is affected and the mother is a carrier, the offspring will have the probability of being one affected female, one affected male, one normal and one carrier female.
- A mother who is a carrier has a 50% chance of passing the faulty X chromosome to her daughter, while an affected father will always pass on the affected gene to his daughters.
- An affected cousin on the mother's side indicates that all women are at risk of being carriers, so their male offspring will be at risk.

- An affected father will pass the gene to his daughters (who become carriers) but will not pass the condition to his sons.
- A female child in an affected family who has Turner syndrome will be at risk (since she has a single X chromosome).

8. e

Isoimmunisation (haemolytic disease of the newborn, erythroblastosis fetalis), antibodies to red cell antigens including Rh, ABO, Duffy and Kell. Anti-Kell antibodies do not affect haemolysis but rather influence red cell production; therefore, amniocentesis is not reliable in monitoring the disease. The critical antibody level is 4 IU/mL.

The mirror syndrome is seen in hydrops fetalis, when the mother develops pre-eclampsia and the severity of her condition 'mirrors' that of the foetus. Doppler umbilical (not uterine) artery waveforms may provide guidance in the diagnosis of foetal anaemia. Middle cerebral artery Doppler waveforms accurately predict foetal anaemia.

Additional reading

Available at: http://patient.info/doctor/hydrops-fetalis

9. d

Triploidy is mostly caused by dispermy or due to fertilisation by diploid sperm. This can lead to partial hydatidiform changes in the placenta. When this results from an additional set of maternal chromosomes, the placenta is small.

Triploid cells contain three sets of the haploid number of chromosomes ($23 \times 3 = 69$). Triploidy is a common finding in spontaneously aborted products of conception. It is rarely seen in live born, and when this happens survival beyond the early neonatal period can occur only in children who are mosaics (cells with diploid and triploid cells).

10. d

Autosomal dominant inheritance refers to conditions caused by changes in the genes located on the autosomes (22 pairs). They occur in both women and men and are not related to whether the foetus is male or female.

Additional reading

Available at: http://www.kumc.edu/AMA-MSS/Study/table_of_genetic_disorders.
   htm
Available at: http://www.geneticalliance.org.uk/docs/translations/english/1-dom-
   he-t.pdf

11. c
Fanconi anaemia is an autosomal recessive condition.

Autosomal dominant inheritance
Both homozygous and heterozygous individuals for the mutant allele will be affected in people who have autosomal dominant inherited conditions. The offspring of an individual with this condition has a one in two (50%) chance of being affected. Often it is possible to trace the disorder through generations in the family, and this condition affects every generation. Autosomal dominant inheritance conditions are as follows: • Adult polycystic kidney disease • Achondroplasia • Ehlers-Danlos syndrome • Familial hypercholesterolaemia • Familial adenomatous polyposis coli • Gilbert syndrome • Huntington chorea • Neurofibromatosis types 1 and 2 • Tuberose sclerosis • Myotonic dystrophy • Marfan syndrome • Von Hippel-Lindau disease • Von Willebrand disease

12. e

Marfan syndrome is an autosomal dominant condition.

Autosomal recessive inheritance
Autosomal recessive inheritance manifests only in individuals who are homozygous for the mutant allele. Individuals who are heterozygous for the condition often show no features and are completely healthy (carriers).   Autosomal recessive inheritance conditions are as follows: • Ataxia telangiectasia   • Alkaptonuria   • β-Thalassaemia   • Congenital adrenal hyperplasia   • Cystic fibrosis   • Dubin-Johnson syndrome   • Fanconi anaemia   • Galactosaemia   • G6PD deficiency   • Glycogen storage diseases   • Haemochromatosis   • Homocystinuria   • Oculocutaneous albinism   • Phenylketonuria   • Tay-Sachs disease   • Spinal muscular atrophy   • Sickle cell anaemia   • Wilson disease

REPRODUCTIVE MEDICINE OR SUBFERTILITY

Questions

1. A 29-year-old woman is referred to the infertility clinic. The couple is seen together in the clinic. She is reviewed with the following investigations:

   - Midcycle progesterone is 65 ng/mL
   - Normal day 3 follicle-stimulating hormone (FSH) and luteinising hormone (LH)
   - Normal hysterosalpingo-contrast-sonography (HyCoSy) scan
   - Normal thyroid function
   - Normal serum prolactin
   - Transvaginal scan – Normal
   - Semen analysis – Azoospermia

   The semen analysis is repeated 3 months later which still shows azoospermia.

   The following can cause azoospermia except one condition. Which one is the exception?
   a. Cystic fibrosis carrier
   b. Kallmann syndrome
   c. Testosterone therapy
   d. Klinefelter syndrome
   e. Down syndrome

2. A 28-year-old woman is referred to infertility clinic. She has been trying to conceive for the last 2 years.

   Which one of the following is a recognised indication for ovum donation treatment in her case?
   a. Turner syndrome
   b. Kallmann syndrome
   c. Androgen-insensitivity syndrome
   d. Rokitansky syndrome
   e. Congenital adrenal hyperplasia

3. A 35-year-old woman presents to the GP with primary infertility. She has been trying to conceive for the last year but has not been successful. She also complains of hot flushes and irritability for the last 3 months. Her FSH is 60 IU/mL. A provisional diagnosis of premature ovarian failure has been made.

Which of the following in her case yields the best pregnancy rate?
a. Ovulation induction
b. Spontaneous sporadic conception
c. Ovum donation
d. Ovarian transposition
e. Ovarian biopsy

4. A 40-year-old woman attends early pregnancy unit at 10 weeks for vaginal spotting. She is due to have her dating scan at 13 weeks of gestation.

Which of the following is not a risk factor for having a twin pregnancy?
a. IVF
b. Older age
c. Personal history of monochorionic twins
d. Maternal family history of dizygotic twins
e. Japanese origin

5. A 40-year-old woman has been trying to conceive for the last 2 years but has not been successful. She had one failed IVF cycle and is going for a second cycle of IVF treatment.

Which of the following will not reduce the success rate of IVF pregnancy?
a. Rising age
b. Previous unsuccessful IVF cycle
c. Body mass index (BMI) 35
d. Consumption of less than one unit of alcohol twice a week
e. Smoking

6. A 35-year-old woman has been trying to conceive for the last 2 years. She and her husband underwent all the investigations and they have been reported normal. She has been counselled to have artificial insemination.

Which one of the following is not true regarding the success rate of artificial insemination?
a. Over 50% of women under the age of 40 years will conceive within six cycles of intrauterine insemination (IUI).
b. The use of fresh sperm is associated with a higher conception rate with intracervical insemination compared to IUI.
c. The use of fresh sperm is associated with a higher conception rate than frozen-thawed sperm.
d. The use of frozen-thawed sperm is associated with a higher conception rate with IUI compared to intracervical insemination.
e. Of the women who do not conceive within the first six cycles of artificial insemination, 50% will do so with a further six cycles.

7. The GP has referred a 26-year-old woman to the infertility clinic who has been trying to conceive for the last 2 years. Her pelvic ultrasound is normal. Her husband has fathered a child from his previous relationship. His semen analysis is as follows with the referral form.

Which one of the following parameters is an abnormal result?
a. Percentage of abnormal form: 85%
b. Progressive motility: 35%
c. pH: 7.12
d. Total sperm number: 40 million
e. Semen volume: 2 mL

8. A 42-year-old woman is undergoing IVF treatment at the IVF centre. She is attending her follow-up appointment after being on the gonadotrophin stimulation protocol. She had various tests to test her response to treatment.

Which one of the following results indicates a higher response to gonadotrophin stimulation?
a. Oestradiol level 266 IU/L
b. FSH 9 IU/L for a high response
c. Anti-müllerian hormone of 25.5 pmol/L
d. Ovarian volume of 15 cc
e. Total antral follicle count of 4

9. A 30-year-old Asian woman is referred to the fertility clinic. She has been trying to conceive for the last 14 months. Her recent HyCoSy scan reveals a normal uterine cavity and tubes. A day 21 serum progesterone level is reported to be 31 ng/mL. Her husband's semen analysis results are reported as follows:
Percentage of abnormal form: 85%
Progressive motility: 35%
pH: 7.22
Total sperm number: 40 million
Semen volume: 2 mL

How should she be managed regarding her subfertility?
a. IVF with intra-cytoplasmic sperm injection (ICSI)
b. Clomiphene citrate for three cycles followed by IUI
c. Clomiphene citrate and IUI
d. Advise regular unprotected intercourse at least three times a week
e. Clomiphene citrate for six cycles followed by IUI

10. A 38-year-old Asian woman has been referred to the infertility clinic. She has been trying to conceive for the last 2 years with her menstrual cycles every 6 weeks. Her ultrasound scan shows two small intramural fibroids and two large subserosal fibroids and polycystic ovaries. Her husband's semen analysis is normal. A recent HyCoSy scan of the uterine cavity and tubes is normal. Her serum progesterone level is reported to be 20 ng/mL. She smokes five cigarettes per day and her BMI is 35. She has one child from her previous partner. She wants to discuss her current options for IVF treatment.

What would be the next course of management in her case?
a. Laparoscopic myomectomy
b. Clomiphene citrate for six cycles
c. Clomiphene citrate for six cycles with IUI after three cycles
d. Lifestyle modifications and advise weight loss
e. Offer IVF as she has been trying for 2 years

Answers

1. e

AZOOSPERMIA (ABSENCE OF THE SPERM FROM THE EJACULATE)

Causes of azoospermia

Pre-testicular	Testicular	Post-testicular
Congenital Hypogonadotrophic hypogonadism (e.g. Kallmann syndrome)	Congenital Klinefelter syndrome (47XXY or Y chromosome deletion)	Obstructive Congenital Bilateral congenital absence of vas deferens (associated with cystic fibrosis in 70%) Acquired Following infection or surgery (e.g. mumps, tubercular epididymitis)
Acquired Testicular trauma Testicular tumour Testosterone therapy	Acquired Previous chemotherapy Previous radiotherapy	Non-obstructive Diabetic nephropathy Prostatectomy (can result in retrograde ejaculation)
	Idiopathic	
	This causes either testicular dysfunction or testicular failure	One should rule out the faulty technique in collection or inadequate sample; therefore, the semen analysis has to be repeated to confirm azoospermia before further investigation
In obstructive azoospermia, the sperm can be aspirated from the vas deferens and used for *in vitro* fertilisation (IVF).		

Additional reading

Bader, T. *OB/GYN Secrets*. 3rd ed. Maryland Heights: Mosby, 2004.
Collins, S et al. *Oxford Handbook of Obstetrics and Gynaecology*. 3rd ed. Oxford: Oxford University Press; 2013.

2. a

Egg donation is required when the woman cannot produce her own eggs, or has poor quality eggs which are unlikely to lead to a successful pregnancy, or she may be carrying a genetic disease that she does not wish to risk transmitting to her children. Kallmann and congenital adrenal hyperplasia are treated with various medications. The uterus is absent in androgen insensitivity and Rokitansky syndrome. Egg donation with surrogacy is required in the former case; while in the latter surrogacy with the patient's own eggs could be used.

Additional reading

National Institute for Health and Care Excellence (NICE). Fertility problems: Assessment and treatment. NICE guidelines (CG156). February 2013.

3. c

Premature ovarian failure is a loss of ovarian function before the age of 45 years. In premature ovarian failure, the ovaries stop producing normal levels of oestrogen and may not produce eggs. It affects about one in 100 women before the age of 40 and five in 100 women before the age of 45.

Around 5%–10% of women will have sporadic ovulation and therefore should be advised to use contraception to avoid pregnancy if they have already completed their family.

Causes of premature ovarian failure

- Idiopathic
- Autoimmune
- Congenital: chromosomal, metabolic
- Immunologic

Iatrogenic causes include surgery, radiotherapy and chemotherapy.

Diagnosis of premature ovarian failure

- History and examination.
- Women with premature ovarian failure usually have raised FSH levels and low levels of oestradiol. FSH and LH should be measured twice at least 5–6 weeks apart.

Management of premature ovarian failure

- Hormone replacement therapy for vaso-motor symptoms, end-organ atrophy and prevention of osteoporosis

Chances of fertility in women with premature ovarian failure

- About 25%–30% pregnancy rate per cycle with oocyte donation.
- Sporadically 1% chance of spontaneous pregnancy/year. (In premature ovarian failure, the function of the ovaries can return intermittently and some women may even start to have periods or become pregnant many years later, although this is rare.)

- Women with idiopathic premature ovarian failure do sometimes ovulate, and approximately 5%–10% will become pregnant over their lifetimes.
- Ovulation induction is not useful.

Additional reading

NICE guidance: Menopause diagnosis and management (NG23). November 2015. http://www.nice.org.uk/guidance/ng23/chapter/Recommendations# managing-short-term-menopausal-symptoms

4. c

Monozygotic twins (identical twins) form from a single zygote that splits after fertilization. They are always of the same gender. Dizygotic twins (fraternal twins) are twins formed from fertilization of two separate eggs by two separate sperms. If more than two eggs are released and fertilized with sperms it becomes mutizygotic twins and this can be triplets, quadruplets, quintuplets, sextuplets, septuplets and octuplets.

Reasons for twins

- The reason for monozygotic twins is not explained. Its incidence is stable across the world.
- Dizygotic twins are more common in older women and probably this is due to release of more than one egg during ovulation (hyperovulate). Women over 30 years of age and more so after 35 years of age.
- Invitro-fertilisation treatment.
- Ovulation inducing drugs.
- Family history of twins.
- Taller women are more likely to have twins.
- Women of African descent are more likely to have twins than Asian descent.

Additional reading

Available at: http://www.motherandbaby.co.uk/trying-for-a-baby/pregnancy-planning/help-to-get-pregnant/6-factors-that-increase-your-chance-of-having-twins-or-multiple-babies
https://www.verywell.com/causes-of-twins-2447133

5. d

The following factors will reduce the success rates of IVF treatment:

- Rising female age
- Number of previous unsuccessful cycles
- BMI outside the range of 19–30
- Consumption of more than one unit of alcohol per day
- Maternal and paternal smoking
- Maternal consumption of caffeine (evidence not consistent)

IVF treatment is more effective in women who had live birth before and/or had previously been pregnant.

Additional reading

National Institute for Health and Care Excellence (NICE). Fertility problems: Assessment and treatment. NICE guidelines (CG156), February 2013. http://www.nice.org.uk/guidance/cg156/chapter/1-recommendations#prediction-of-ivf-success

6. b

SUCCESS WITH IUI

- Over 50% of women under the age of 40 years will conceive within six cycles of IUI.
- Of the women who do not conceive within the first six cycles of artificial insemination, 50% will do so with a further six cycles (cumulative pregnancy rate of 75%).
- Even when frozen-thawed sperm are used, IUI is associated with a higher pregnancy rate than intracervical insemination.

Additional reading

National Institute for Health and Care Excellence (NICE). Fertility problems: Assessment and treatment. NICE guidelines (CG156). February 2013. http://www.nice.org.uk/guidance/cg156/chapter/1-recommendations#prediction-of-ivf-success

7. c

REFERENCE VALUES

The results of the semen analysis conducted as part of an initial assessment should be compared with the following World Health Organization (WHO) reference values:

- Semen volume: 1.5 mL or more
- pH: 7.2 or more
- Sperm concentration: 15 million spermatozoa per millilitre or more
- Total sperm number: 39 million spermatozoa per ejaculate or more
- Total motility (percentage of progressive motility and non-progressive motility): 40% or more motile or 32% or more with progressive motility
- Vitality: 58% or more live spermatozoa
- Sperm morphology (percentage of normal forms): 4% or more

Additional reading

National Institute for Health and Care Excellence (NICE). Fertility problems: Assessment and treatment. NICE guidelines (CG156), February 2013. https://www.nice.org.uk/guidance/qs73/chapter/quality-statement-4-semen-analysis

8. c

Ovarian response to gonadotrophin stimulation in IVF is measured by use of one of the following parameters:

- Total antral follicle count of ≤ 4 for a low response and >16 for a high response
- Anti-müllerian hormone of ≤ 5.4 pmol/L for a low response and ≥ 25 pmol/L for a high response
- FSH >8.9 IU/L for a low response and <4 IU/L for a high response

Additional reading

National Institute for Health and Care Excellence (NICE). Fertility problems: Assessment and treatment. NICE guidelines (CG156), February 2013. http://www.nice.org.uk/guidance/cg156/chapter/1-recommendations

9. d

Additional reading

National Institute for Health and Care Excellence (NICE). Fertility problems: Assessment and treatment. NICE guidelines (CG156), February 2013. http://www.nice.org.uk/guidance/cg156/chapter/1-recommendations

10. d

OBESITY

- Women who have a BMI of 30 or over should be informed that they are likely to take longer to conceive.
- Women who have a BMI of 30 or over and who are not ovulating should be informed that losing weight is likely to increase their chance of conception.
- Women should be informed that participating in a group programme involving exercise and dietary advice leads to more pregnancies than weight loss advice alone.
- Men who have a BMI of 30 or over should be informed that they are likely to have reduced fertility.

LOW BODY WEIGHT

- Women who have a BMI of less than 19 and who have irregular menstruation or are not menstruating should be advised that increasing body weight is likely to improve their chance of conception.

Additional reading

National Institute for Health and Care Excellence (NICE). Fertility problems: Assessment and treatment. NICE guidelines (CG156), February 2013. http://www.nice.org.uk/guidance/cg156/chapter/1-recommendations

SURGICAL PROCEDURES AND CORE SURGICAL SKILLS

Questions

1. A 20-year-old woman presents to the early pregnancy assessment unit with abdominal pain. An ultrasound scan reveals left tubal ectopic pregnancy of 3.5×3 cm. She undergoes laparoscopy and the findings are as follows:

   Left tubal unruptured ectopic pregnancy of 3 cm with normal right fallopian tube. Minimal endometriosis in the pouch of Douglas with extensive bowel adhesions on the right side due to previous appendisectomy. Uterus is bulky but normal.

   How should she be managed?
   a. Left salpingostomy with treatment of endometriosis
   b. Left salpingectomy with adhesiolysis
   c. Left salpingostomy with adhesiolysis and treatment of endometriosis
   d. Left salpingectomy
   e. Abandon laparoscopy and treat with medical management (methotrexate)

2. A 25-year-old woman attends the emergency department with a history of left-sided severe abdominal pain for the last 24 hours. A clinical diagnosis of suspected ovarian torsion is made as there is marked tenderness as well as guarding on abdominal palpation. An ultrasound scan reveals a large ovarian dermoid cyst on the left side ($9 \times 7 \times 8$ cm) with absent blood flow. Bloods reveal leucocytosis and raised C-reactive protein. A laparotomy is performed in view of clinical suspicions of ovarian torsion.

   Intra-operative findings reveal the following:

   - Normal right ovary
   - Torsion of ovarian pedicle $\times$ 3 loops (left ovary)
   - Left ovary appears non-viable
   - Normal fallopian tubes and uterus
   - Normal rest of pelvis and abdomen with no ascites

   Her surgical management includes which one of the following?
   a. Left salpingo-oophorectomy
   b. Left salpingectomy and left ovarian cystectomy
   c. Left ovarian cystectomy
   d. Left-sided oophorectomy
   e. Left-sided oophorectomy and peritoneal washings

3. A 38-year-old woman, para 1, presents to the labour ward at 41 weeks of gestation with regular contractions every 3 minutes. Abdominal examination reveals ballotable head and vaginal examination reveals early labour. An hour later, she has a spontaneous rupture of membranes and cord prolapse. She is pushed to theatre for crash caesarean section. What is her risk of bladder injury?
   a. 4–6/10,000
   b. 1/1000
   c. 3/1000
   d. 5/1000
   e. 1–2/100

4. A 36-year-old woman had a normal vaginal delivery when she was 20 years old (for maternal request). She is now 30 weeks' pregnant and wants a repeat elective caesarean section. What are her chances of death if she has a planned cesarean section at 39 weeks of gestation?
   a. 15/100,000
   b. 13/100,000
   c. 11/100,000
   d. 5/100,000
   e. 1/100,000

5. A 15-year-old girl presents to the early assessment unit at 9 weeks of gestation with mild vaginal bleeding. An ultrasound scan reveals a missed miscarriage. The on-call doctor discusses pros and cons of medical versus surgical management with her. This girl prefers surgical management.

   What would be her risk of uterine perforation?
   a. Up to 2/1000
   b. Up to 4/1000
   c. Up to 5/1000
   d. Up to 3/100
   e. Up to 1/100

6. An 18-year-old woman comes with abdominal pain to the gynaecology emergency unit. A clinical examination reveals tender abdomen. An ultrasound scan of pelvis is normal. Clinically there are no signs of infection. She was taken to theatre for diagnostic laparoscopy. A Veress needle was inserted for gas insufflation.

   What is the recommended pressure for port insertion?
   a. 10 mm of Hg
   b. 15 mm of Hg
   c. 20 mm of Hg
   d. 25 mm of Hg
   e. 30 mm of Hg

7. An 18-year-old woman comes with abdominal pain to the gynaecology emergency unit. A clinical examination reveals tender abdomen. An ultrasound scan of pelvis is normal. Clinically there are no signs of infection.

She was taken to theatre for diagnostic laparoscopy. She had one suprapubic 7 mm port, one 10 mm umbilical port and one lateral 7 mm port on the left side and one lateral 5 mm port on the right side.

Which of the following port sites rectus sheath should be closed with Vicryl 1?
a. All port sites
b. 7 mm lateral port, 7 mm suprapubic port and 10 mm umbilical port
c. 7 mm suprapubic port and 10 mm umbilical port
d. 7 mm lateral port and 5 mm lateral port
e. Only 10 mm umbilical port

8. A 56-year-old woman has a staging laparotomy for stage 3 ovarian cancer.

The following measures improve the best possible outcome with regards to abdominal incisions except for one. Which statement is the exception?
a. Making a transverse suprapubic skin incision has cosmetic advantages compared with longitudinal incisions but may not allow adequate access
b. A subcuticular suture also improves the cosmetic appearance and enhances postoperative comfort
c. Longitudinal incisions (particularly midline) are more likely to be complicated by the development of wound dehiscence and incisional hernia
d. Mass closure of longitudinal incisions reduces the risk of complete abdominal wound dehiscence and incisional hernia
e. Closure of peritoneal surfaces decreases the risk of intestinal obstruction resulting from adhesions

9. A senior midwife calls you to the delivery suite. A primigravida during a normal delivery sustains a perineal tear.

Which of the following statements is incorrect regarding the degree of perineal tears?
a. First degree – injury to the perineum involving just the skin
b. First degree – injury to the perineum involving both skin and the transverse perineal muscle
c. Second degree – injury to the perineum not involving the anal sphincter
d. Third degree – injury to the perineum involving the anal sphincter complex
e. Fourth degree – injury to the perineum involving the rectal mucosa

10. A 40-year-old para 2 woman is referred to the gynaecology clinic for menorrhagia. She has an outpatient hysteroscopy and Pipelle biopsy which is normal. She has tried Mirena but this has not reduced her bleeding. She undergoes a NovaSure endometrial ablation.

Which one of the following expectations might not be met?
a. Dysmenorrhoea might not be relieved
b. Premenstrual syndrome might not be relieved
c. Subsequent pregnancy is not contraindicated
d. Successful reduction in bleeding occurred in 98% of the patients by 12 months
e. Subsequent contraception will not be required

Answers

1. d

A laparoscopic approach to the surgical management of tubal pregnancy, in the haemodynamically stable patient, is preferable to an open approach.

Management of tubal pregnancy in the presence of haemodynamic instability should be by the most expedient method. In most cases this will be laparotomy.

In the presence of a healthy contralateral tube, salpingectomy should be used instead of salpingotomy. This approach is associated with a lower rate of persistent trophoblast and subsequent tubal ectopic pregnancies while achieving similar intrauterine pregnancy rates.

Laparoscopic salpingotomy should be considered as the primary treatment when managing tubal pregnancy in the presence of contralateral tubal disease and the desire for future fertility. The woman should be warned about the risk of persistent trophoblast and the 20% risk of ectopic pregnancy with salpingostomy.

Non-sensitised women who are Rhesus negative with a confirmed or suspected ectopic pregnancy, managed medically or surgically, should receive anti-D immunoglobulin.

An increased risk of recurrence in future pregnancies (10%) should be explained and the need for an early scan (at 6 weeks) in future pregnancies should be emphasised.

Additional reading

Magowan B. *Churchill's Pocketbook of Obstetrics and Gynaecology.* 3rd ed. Edinburgh: Churchill Livingston, 2005.

Royal College of Obstetricians and Gynaecologists (RCOG). *Green-top Guideline No. 21. Management of Tubal Pregnancy.* London: RCOG Press, 2004.

Stovall TG, Ling FW, Carson SA, Buster JE. Serum progesterone and uterine curettage in differential diagnosis of ectopic pregnancy. *Fertility and Sterility.* 1992;57:456–7. https://www.ncbi.nlm.nih.gov/pubmed/1735503

2. e

OVARIAN CYST ACCIDENTS

Ovarian accidents include ovarian cyst rupture, ovarian cyst torsion and haemorrhage into the ovarian cyst.

Ovarian cyst rupture and haemorrhage usually occur in association with physiological functional cysts and are generally self-limiting.

Ovarian torsion is defined as partial or complete rotation of the ovarian vascular pedicle. The majority of ovarian cyst torsion occurs in the reproductive age but about one-quarter of cases occur in children.

An ovarian mass has been found in 64%–82% of cases of confirmed torsion. The size of the cyst is usually 6 cm or more (moderate size) with long pedicles. Cysts of this size are usually lifted over the confines of the pelvis and become more freely mobile. It is postulated that a heavy ovary allows the ovary to swing on its pedicle. The tube and ovary usually undergo torsion as a single unit, rotating around the broad ligament as an axis. Commonly, the ovary twists alone, around the mesovarium. In the absence of an ovarian cyst, the torsion occurs where there is an unusually long pedicle. This causes occlusion of the venous return followed later by occlusion of the arterial inflow to the ovarian tumour. An ultrasound scan shows an oedematous ovary with peripheral displacement of the follicles.

Ovarian torsions occur twice as often with the right adnexa than with the left adnexa suggesting anatomic differences such as the presence of the sigmoid colon (it restricts the mobility of the left ovary). In accordance with Kushner's rule, the right ovary twists in a clockwise manner and the left counterclockwise.

Mature cystic teratomas are common tumours leading to torsion (3.5%–10% of them undergo torsion), followed by cystadenomas, dysfunctional cysts, ovarian hyperstimulation, polycystic ovaries and para-ovarian cysts. It is less common in women with endometriosis, previous pelvic inflammatory disease (PID) or malignancy (2% of the ovarian malignancies undergo torsion) as these are relatively fixed in the pelvis and therefore less mobile.

Management

Most cases of ovarian torsion require surgical intervention except in mild and early cases where there is the possibility of untwisting naturally.

This woman should be managed surgically and the approach can be laparotomy or laparoscopy. This depends on the availability of expertise.

The aim should be fertility-sparing surgery where possible in young women. If the ovarian tissue can be preserved (if the ovary appears viable), an ovarian cystectomy should be performed, while unilateral oophorectomy is considered in the worst case scenario where the ovary is non-viable.

Following surgery, debriefing is very important. This woman should be followed up in the clinic to discuss the histology results.

She should be informed that her fertility is unlikely to be affected.

Additional reading

Bottomley C, Bourne T. Diagnosis and management of ovarian cyst accidents. *Best Practice and Research: Clinical Obstetrics and Gynaecology.* 2009;23:711–24.

3. b

RISKS OF CAESAREAN SECTION

Serious risks: Maternal

- Emergency hysterectomy, 7–8 women in every 1000 undergoing caesarian section
- Need for further surgery at a later date, including curettage, 5 in 1000 women
- Admission to intensive care unit (highly dependent on the reason for caesarean section), 9 in 1000 women
- Thromboembolic disease, 4–16 in 10,000 women
- Bladder injury, 1 in 1000 women
- Ureteric injury, 3 in 10,000 women
- Death, approximately 1 in 12,000 women

Frequent risks: Maternal

- Persistent wound and abdominal discomfort in the first few months after surgery, 9 in 100 women
- Increased risk of a repeat caesarean section when vaginal delivery is attempted in subsequent pregnancies, 1 in 4 women
- Readmission to hospital, 5 in 100 women
- Haemorrhage, 5 in 1000 women
- Infection, 6 in 100 women

Frequent risk: Fetal

- Lacerations, 1–2 in 100 babies

Risks for future pregnancies

- Increased risk of uterine rupture during subsequent pregnancies/deliveries, 2–7 in 1000 women
- Increased risk of antepartum stillbirth, 2–4 in 1000 women
- Increased risk of placenta praevia and placenta accreta, 4–8 in 1000 women

Additional procedures during caesarean section which may become necessary include hysterectomy, repair of injured organs and blood transfusion.

Additional reading

Royal College of Obstetricians and Gynaecologists. *Consent Advice No. 7. Caesarean Section*. London: RCOG Press, 2009.

Royal College of Obstetricians and Gynaecologists. *Green-top Guideline No. 45. Birth After Previous Caesarean Section*. London: RCOG Press, October 2015.

RISKS AND BENEFITS OF PLANNED CAESAREAN SECTION

- Risk of transient respiratory morbidity of 4%–5% (6% risk if delivery performed at 38 instead of 39 weeks). The risk is reduced with antenatal corticosteroids, but there are concerns about potential long-term adverse effects.
- Less than 1 per 10,000 (<0.01%) risk of delivery-related perinatal death or hypoxic ischemic encephalopathy (HIE).
- Virtually avoids the risk of uterine rupture (actual risk is extremely low: less than 0.02%).
- Reduces the risk of pelvic organ prolapse and urinary incontinence in comparison with number of vaginal births (dose-response effect) at least in the short term.
- Option for sterilisation if fertility is no longer desired. Evidence suggests that the regret rate is higher and that the failure rate from sterilisation associated with pregnancy may be higher than that from an interval procedure. If sterilisation is to be performed at the same time as a caesarean delivery, counselling and agreement should have been given at least 2 weeks prior to the procedure.
- Future pregnancies – likely to require caesarean delivery, increased risk of placenta praevia/accreta and adhesions with successive caesarean deliveries/abdominal surgery.

Additional reading

Royal College of Obstetricians and Gynaecologists. *Green-top Guideline No. 45. Birth After Previous Caesarean Section.* London: RCOG Press, October 2015.
Royal College of Obstetricians and Gynaecologists. *Consent Advice No. 7. Caesarean Section.* London: RCOG Press, 2009.

5. c

SURGICAL EVACUATION OF UTERUS (EVACUATION OF RETAINED PRODUCTS OF CONCEPTION [ERPC])

Serious risks include the following:

- Uterine perforation, up to 5 in 1000 women
- Significant trauma to the cervix

There is no substantiated evidence in the literature of any impact on future fertility.

Frequent risks include the following:

- Bleeding that lasts for up to 2 weeks is very common but blood transfusion is uncommon (1–2 in 1000 women).
- Need for repeat surgical evacuation, up to 5 in 100 women
- Localised pelvic infection, 3 in 100 women

The additional procedures that may be necessary during the procedure include laparoscopy or laparotomy to diagnose or repair organ injury, or uterine perforation.

Additional reading

Royal College of Obstetricians and Gynaecologists. *Consent Advice No. 10. Surgical Evacuation of Uterus for Early Pregnancy Loss*. London: RCOG Press, 2010.

6. c

Additional reading

StratOG: The RCOGs online learning.

7. c

DIAGNOSTIC LAPAROSCOPY

- Place the patient in Lloyd Davies position and flat on table.
- Empty the bladder before operation.
- Check the Verres for gas flow and spring action.
- White balance and focus the scope.
- Double click.
- Make vertical umbilical incision at the base of the umbilicus.
- Conduct a Palmer test.
- Ensure Verres is inserted perpendicular to the skin surface.
- Confirm entry pressure <8 mm Hg.
- Once abdominal cavity is entered do not move the Verres needle sideways as a small bowel perforation can become large.
- Perform gas insufflation until the pressure is 20 mm Hg. Warn the anaesthetist.
- Take the Verres out and insert 5 or 10 mm port perpendicular to the umbilicus.

- Insert the laparoscope and take a 360° look to make sure you have not injured any vessel or bowel.
- If everything is all right attach the gas lead to the umbilical port.
- Look for landmarks inside the abdomen before inserting secondary ports.
- Check median umbilical ligament obliterated umbilical ligaments and inferior epigastric artery.
- Note that inferior epigastric artery is lateral to the obliterated umbilical ligaments.
- Ensure all the secondary ports are lateral to inferior epigastric arteries.
- Note that all secondary ports should be inserted under direct vision before the Trendelenburg position is asked (can be lateral or midline suprapubic in position).
- Ask for head low and get the pressures down to 15 mm Hg.
- Do a systematic examination of the pelvis (e.g. from left to right side including ovarian fossa, lateral pelvic wall, pouch of Douglas and uterovesical fold of peritoneum and liver).
- Level the table once the procedure is complete.
- Remove all ports under direct vision (look for port site bleeding before ports are removed).
- Expel gas as it can cause severe postoperative abdominal and shoulder pain.
- Inject local to port sites.
- Close the rectus sheath with suture Vicryl 1 (if midline incisions are 7 mm or more and lateral incisions 10 mm or more).
- Remove the vaginal instruments and do an instrument count.

Additional reading

Royal College of Obstetricians and Gynaecologists. *Green-top Guideline No. 2. Diagnostic Laparoscopy*. London: RCOG Press, 2008.

8. e

PRINCIPLES OF SURGICAL CARE

- Optimising the patient's preoperative condition may improve outcome (e.g. reduction in smoking, giving chest physio, weight reduction, anaemia, ensuring no infections)
- The site and extent of the incision, which may be longitudinal, transverse or (seldom) oblique, should be appropriate for the nature and purpose of the operation.
- Making a transverse suprapubic skin incision has cosmetic advantages compared with longitudinal incisions but may not allow adequate access.
- A subcuticular suture also improves the cosmetic appearance and enhances postoperative comfort.

- Longitudinal incisions (particularly midline) are more likely to be complicated by the development of wound dehiscence and incisional hernia.
- Mass closure of longitudinal incisions reduces the risk of complete abdominal wound dehiscence and incisional hernia.
- Closure of peritoneal surfaces may increase the risk of intestinal obstruction resulting from adhesions.
- Prophylactic antibiotics are effective in reducing the risk of wound infection but rigorous discipline in antiseptic techniques, limiting wound contamination and fastidious haemostasis remain fundamentally important.
- Wound drains reduce the risk of wound haematoma especially in women given prophylactic anticoagulant therapy.
- Non-absorbable sutures are associated with a lower risk of wound dehiscence (catgut is no longer used in the United Kingdom).

Additional reading

StratOG: The RCOGs online learning.

9. b

If the tear is thought to be third or fourth degree or is unable to be fully assessed, then

- Repair of the defect needs to be undertaken in an operating theatre under regional or general anaesthesia and by an experienced surgeon.
- It is advised to use a monofilament suture to repair the defect as this is associated with a lower infection rate and better long-term function.
- There is no clear-cut evidence of benefit for either overlapping or end-to-end approximation technique of repair of anal sphincter.
- Prophylactic broad-spectrum antibiotic should be used during and after repair of anal sphincter.
- Offer a follow-up appointment with a gynaecologist with an interest in anorectal dysfunction. If the patient is symptomatic at follow-up, an endo-anal ultrasound or a rectal manometry should be arranged prior to a secondary repair by a surgeon with appropriate expertise.
- One should discuss the option of abdominal delivery in future pregnancies if the patient remains symptomatic.

Additional reading

StratOG: The RCOGs online learning. https://stratog.rcog.org. uk/tutorial/management-of-postoperative-complications/ investigation-of-the-renal-tract-586

10. d

Amenorrhea rates for the NovaSure procedure ranged from 30% to 75%. Patients who reported being satisfied with the NovaSure procedure ranged from 85% to 94%. In randomised controlled trials with other global endometrial ablation modalities, amenorrhea rates at 12 months with the NovaSure procedure ranged from 43% to 56%, while other modalities ranged from 8% to 24%. By 60 months post-procedure, 75% of the patients reported amenorrhea and 2% reported menorrhagia. Only four (3.9%) patients reported menorrhagia at 12 months.

Additional reading

Gimpelson RJ. Ten-year literature review of global endometrial ablation with the NovaSure® device. *International Journal of Women's Health.* 2014;6:269–80. http://www.ncbi.nlm.nih.gov/pmc/articles/PMC3956630/
StratOG: The RCOGs online learning.

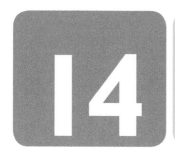

14 POST-OPERATIVE COMPLICATIONS

Questions

1. A 48-year-old woman undergoes laparoscopic hysterectomy and bilateral salpingo-oophorectomy, pelvic lymphadenectomy, peritoneal washings and bowel adhesiolysis for International Federation of Gynecology and Obstetrics (FIGO) stage Ib, high-grade serous endometrial cancer. Her blood loss was 1000 mL. A peritoneal pelvic drain is inserted. Her observations are stable and she is apyrexial. Her abdominal drain is straw-coloured fluid and is 500 mL on day 2. Her haemoglobin (HB) is 9 gm% and serum creatinine is 75. Drain fluid creatinine is reported as 90.

   What is the diagnosis in her case?
   a. Urinoma
   b. Ureteric injury
   c. Ascites
   d. Lymphocele
   e. Pelvic collection

2. A 48-year-old woman undergoes laparoscopic hysterectomy and bilateral salpingo-oophorectomy, pelvic lymphadenectomy and peritoneal washings for grade 3 endometrial cancer. It was a difficult operation due to extensive adhesions. Her abdominal drain is straw-coloured fluid and is 500 mL on day 2. She is clinically stable. Her haemoglobin (HB) is 9 gm% and serum creatinine is 75. Drain fluid creatinine is reported as 90.

   Which of the following is not a sign or symptom of urinary tract injury in her case?
   a. Persistent loin pain
   b. Poor urine output in the presence of normal postoperative observations – urine leaking into peritoneal cavity
   c. Anuria
   d. Urine draining vaginally
   e. Persistent very heavily bloodstained urine postoperatively with later leakage of fluid into the vagina
   f. Only straw colour fluid in the peritoneal drain

3. A 48-year-old woman undergoes hysterectomy and bilateral salpingo-oophorectomy, pelvic lymphadenectomy and peritoneal washings for grade 3

endometrial cancer. You are the registrar on call for gynaecology and have been asked to review this woman whose urine output is 20 mL for the previous 8 hours (day 1 of the operation). The operation notes reveal that this was a difficult operation due to extensive bowel and pelvic adhesions. She has an abdominal drain which is drained 400 mL. Her urine output is 20 mL in the last 8 hours. She is clinically stable. Her haemoglobin (HB) is 12 gm% and serum creatinine is 75. Drain fluid creatinine is reported as 90.

You are suspecting a ureteric injury or occlusion. What is most important investigation that would help in making a diagnosis of ureteric injury or occlusion?

a. Computed tomography (CT) scan pelvis with contrast
b. Magnetic resonance imaging (MRI) scan pelvis with contrast
c. Intravenous urogram
d. Positron emission tomography (PET) scan of kidney, ureter and bladder
e. Cystoscopy and methylene blue test

4. A 48-year-old woman undergoes laparoscopic hysterectomy and bilateral salpingo-oophorectomy, pelvic lymphadenectomy, bowel and pelvic adhesiolysis and peritoneal washings for grade 3 endometrial cancer. While dissecting the pelvic side wall, the consultant notices right ureteric injury close to the bladder edge. The urologist on call has been called for opinion and repair.

What would be recommended management for her surgically?

a. Right ureter repair and ureteric stenting
b. End-to-end anastomosis of the ureter and ureteric stenting
c. Stenting of the ureter
d. Foley catheter for 2 weeks and stenting of the ureter
e. Ureteric re-implantation into the bladder using a psoas hitch to relieve tension of the repair

5. A 44-year-old woman undergoes laparoscopic subtotal hysterectomy for fibroids with a blood loss of 500 mL. On day 2 (36 hours post-operation) she develops abdominal pain and looks pale. Her haemoglobin (HB) is reported as 7.8 gm% (pre-operative HB: 13 gm%). She is clinically stable and apyrexial with good urine output. She herself is an A&E nurse and is asking for blood transfusion. You are the registrar on call and have been asked to review this woman and make a plan of management.

What should be her immediate management?

a. Laparotomy and drainage of pelvic haematoma
b. Intravenous cannulas, blood transfusion ×2 units, antibiotics, withhold Clexane, close monitoring and repeat HB after transfusion
c. Drainage of vault haematoma through the vault
d. Image-guided (CT scan) drainage of haematoma through abdominal drain
e. Laparoscopic drainage of the haematoma

1. d

In her case, she had pelvic lymphadenectomy. It is likely to be lymphocele which is draining through the drain. The drain fluid creatinine level is representative of serum creatinine level and is not significantly higher; therefore, there is no concern of urinoma in this case.

Additional reading

StratOG: The RCOGs online learning.

2. f

The symptoms of ureteric injury can be fever, haematuria, flank pain, abdominal distension, abscess formation, sepsis, peritonitis and ileus, retroperitoneal urinoma, postoperative anuria, urinary leakage through vagina or abdominal wound and secondary hypertension.

The incidence of ureteric damage in gynaecological surgery can be 0.5%–2.5% depending on the underlying condition pathology. With severe endometriosis, 65% of patients could have the ureteric involvement and a further 5.6% can have ureteric stenosis.

The common sites of ureteric damage include the following:

- At the angle of the vagina
- Near the pelvic brim close to the ovarian blood supply

The damage may be direct during the operation or due to avascular necrosis due to compromised vasculature. The former present early (first few days) and the latter may present 7–10 days after the procedure.

If identified early, stenting of the ureter alone can be sufficient to resolve the damage.

Additional reading

StratOG: The RCOGs online learning. https://stratog.rcog.org.uk/uploads/File/ elearn/Management-of-postoperative-complications/Jha_TOG_2004.pdf
Jha S, Aravinthan C, Chan KK. Ureteric injury in obstetric and gynaecological surgery. *Obstetrician and Gynaecologist.* 2011:6(4); 203–208.
http://onlinelibrary.wiley.com/doi/10.1576/toag.6.4.203.27016/pdf

3. c

INVESTIGATIONS FOR URINARY TRACT INJURIES

- Intravenous urogram (IVU): Shows delayed excretion and a dilated ureter at the level of block
- IVU: Shows leak of the contrast outside the ureter with ureteric injury
- Three-swab test: Will help to identify vesico-vaginal fistulae
- Cystoscopy: Useful to diagnose a vesico-vaginal fistula and may show occlusion of the terminal ureter

Additional reading

StratOG: The RCOGs online learning. https://stratog.rcog.org.uk/tutorial/
    management-of-postoperative-complications/investigation-of-the-renal-tract-586

4. e

The ureteric or bladder injury identified during the operation should be repaired at the same time. Urological opinion should be sought for any suspected or obvious ureteric injuries.

RECOMMENDATIONS OF MANAGEMENT FOR URETERIC INJURY

- Ureteric injury at the pelvic brim: Need end-to-end anastomosis
- Ureteric injury near the bladder edge: Need ureteric reimplantation into the bladder using a psoas hitch or bladder flap to relieve tension on the repair

Following the repair, stenting of the ureter at the same time as repair and follow-up with a urologist are advised.

RECOMMENDATIONS OF MANAGEMENT FOR SUSPECTED FISTULA

- Fistula: Insert a urinary Foley catheter immediately as spontaneous repair of the damaged bladder is dependent upon the extent of the urinary leakage.
- Small fistula: Generally managed conservatively by Foley catheter insertion for 7–10 days with antibiotic cover.
- Surgical repair is indicated if catheterisation fails to resolve the leak (the fistula tract must be fully mobilised and the edges debrided). The repair should be performed with absorbable sutures in one or two layers.

Additional reading

Minas V, Gul N, Aust T, Doyle M, Rowlands D. Urinary tract injuries in
    laparoscopic gynaecological surgery; Prevention, recognition and
    management. *The Obstetrician and Gynaecologist.* January 2014;16:19–28.
StratOG: The RCOGs online learning. https://stratog.rcog.org.uk/tutorial/
    management-of-postoperative-complications/investigation-of-the-renal-tract-586
Wijaya T, Lo T-S, Jaili SB, Wu P-Y. The diagnosis and management of ureteric
    injury after laparoscopy. *Gynecology and Minimally Invasive Therapy.*
    2015;4(2), 29.

5. b

Vault haematomas following hysterectomy is one of the complications of this surgery and is not uncommon. Women can present with abdominal pain or low-grade temperature or with vaginal discharge. Clinically most often they may be stable with a low HB. Most patients respond to conservative treatment with antibiotics and avoiding Clexane and non-steroidal anti-inflammatory drugs (NSAIDs). This helps to prevent infection and also possibly avoid further bleeding.

Few patients are likely to need surgery (laparotomy, drainage, wash out and large-bore Robinson drain) if the patient is symptomatic with persistent pain, shows signs of infection or sepsis (raised temperature or rising inflammatory markers) and if there is a significant drop in HB. Often (small collection of the vault), the haematoma can be drained through a vaginal approach (through vault).

Additional reading

StratOG: The RCOGs online learning. https://stratog.rcog.org.uk/tutorial/
    management-of-postoperative-complications-teaching-resource/
    vault-haematoma-7175

INDEX